Dog Anatomy
A Coloring Atlas

Robert A. Kainer, DVM, MS
Professor Emeritus of Anatomy
College of Veterinary Medicine and Biomedical Sciences
Colorado State University
Fort Collins, Colorado

Thomas O. McCracken, MS
Vice President for Research and Development
Visible Productions LLC
Fort Collins, Colorado

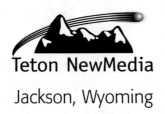
Teton NewMedia

Jackson, Wyoming

Executive Editor: Carroll C. Cann
Development Editor: Susan L. Hunsberger
Editor: Nicol Giandomenico
Art Director and Production Manager: Anita B. Sykes
Design and Layout: 5640 Design, www.fiftysixforty.com
Illustrations by Thomas O. McCracken

Printed in the United States of America

Teton NewMedia
P.O. Box 4833
Jackson, WY 83001

1-888-770-3165
www.tetonnewmedia.com

ISBN# 1-893441-17-2

Print Number 5 4 3

Library of Congress Cataloging-in-Publication Data

Kainer, Robert A.
    A coloring atlas of canine anatomy / Robert A. Kainer, Thomas O. McCracken.
        p. ; cm.
    ISBN 1-893441-17-2
    1. Dogs--Anatomy--Atlases. I. McCracken, Thomas. II. Title.
    [DMLM: 1. Dogs--anatomy & histology--Atlases. 2. Dogs--anatomy &
    histology--Problems and Exercises. SF 767.D6 K13c 2002]
    SF767.D6 K35 2002
    636.7'0891--dc21

Table of Contents

Acknowledgments

The authors express their gratitude to anatomy professors Dr. Michael Smith of Ross University and Dr. Anna Dee Fails of Colorado State University for their critical reviews of the drawings and text. A student's perception and a thorough critique was provided by Mr. Mark Goldstein, dog owner and student of anatomy. Their input assisted substantially in the preparation of this atlas.

The patience and counsel of the staff at Teton New Media is gratefully acknowledged.

Several illustrations were redrawn from the followng sources:

Evans H.E. (ed.): Miller's Anatomy of the Dog, 3rd ed., Philadelphia, W.B. Saunders, l993. Figure 9-7

Noden D.H., deLahunta A.: The Embryology of Domestic Animals, Developmental Mechanisms and Malformations, Baltimore, Williams & Wilkins, 1985. Figure 18-15.

The following publications were used for general reference:

Done S.H., Evans S.A., Strickland N.C.: Color Atlas of Veterinary Anatomy, Vol. 3, The Dog and Cat, London, Mosby-Wolfe, 1996.

Budras K-D., Fricke W., McCarthy P.H.: Anatomy of the Dog – An Illustrated Text, 3rd Ed., London, Mosby-Wolfe,1994.

Evans H.E., (ed.): Miller's Anatomy of the Dog, 3rd Ed., Philadelphia, W.B. Saunders, 1993.

Boyd J.S.: A Color Atlas of Clinical Anatomy of the Dog and Cat, London, Mosby-Wolfe, 1991.

Popesko P.: Atlas of Topographical Anatomy of the Domestic Animals, Philadelphia, W. B. Saunders,1979.

Ellenberger W., Dittrich H., Baum H., Brown L.S. (ed.): An Atlas of Animal Anatomy for Artists, New York, Dover Publications, 1956.

Introduction

This coloring atlas was produced for those with a genuine interest in dogs. The format is designed for the dog owner who desires to gain a basic knowledge of canine anatomy with functional correlations and brief descriptions of some of the diseases of the region being studied. Dog breeders, trainers, and dog show judges as well as students of veterinary medicine, veterinary medical technology, zoology, and wildlife biology will find the contents useful for an initial background from which more detailed references can be pursued. Active learning is involved as you color anatomical structures and their names on the drawings or underline their names in the text and color the parts indicated by a corresponding number. Guiding symbols such as arrows or lines are also colored. As you color, the size, shape, and position of organs and their relationships are made clear.

The dog, *Canis familiaris* (genus species), is a mammal in the order Carnivora and family Canidae. Based on the family name, a dog is a **canid**. The adjective canine is commonly, but erroneously, used as a noun to designate a dog. The word dog is used both as a noun and an adjective. The coyote and the various wolves and jackals are wild canids in the genus *Canis*. Dogs are believed to be descended from several subspecies of wolf in various parts of the world. Closely related to the genus *Canis* are the genera *Vulpes* (foxes) and *Dusicyon* (South American foxes). African wild dogs, *Lycaon* pictus, are more distantly related canids.

Some physical characteristics of canids:
Prominent canine and premolar teeth for holding and cutting skin and flesh.
Carnassial (shearing) teeth – lower first molar and upper fourth premolar teeth.
A relatively short digestive tract.
Anal sacs lined with sebaceous (oil) glands.
Reproductive system producing several offspring in one gestation.
Heart, lungs, and muscular appendages adapted for running or digging.
Nonretractable claws.

Among the approximately 400 breeds of dogs in the world (more than 150 currently recognized by the American Kennel Club), there are many different sizes, shapes, and hair coats. Dogs range in size from 6 inches to 3.5 feet in height and weigh from 2 to over 200 pounds. Whether a dog has the proportions of a Mastiff, a Greyhound, a Boston Terrier, or a Chihuahua, the basic anatomy and physiology are very similar. In this atlas, you will explore the anatomy of the dog and some of the more remarkable variations among the different breeds.

The Authors

Robert A. Kainer, DVM, MS
Professor of Anatomy
College of Veterinary Medicine and Biomedical Sciences
Colorado State University, Fort Collins, Colorado
After receiving his DVM degree from Colorado A & M College (now CSU) in 1949, Dr. Kainer spent a summer at the University of Idaho, then four years at Washington State University where he taught anatomy and pursued graduate study in anatomy and pathology. He was granted a Master of Science degree in veterinary medicine from Washington State. For the next two years, he taught at Oklahoma State University. He returned to Colorado in 1955 to enter private veterinary practice in Idaho Springs. While in practice, he also served as a high school science teacher. In 1961, he joined the anatomy faculty at Colorado State University. Among the honors he received during his 27 years at Colorado State are the Top Prof Award and the Oliver Pennock Award for teaching and scholarship at CSU, the Norden Award for distinguished teaching in the field of veterinary medicine, and the Colorado Veterinary Medical Association 1986 Faculty of the Year Award. Dr. Kainer has contributed his expertise in collaborative research on various veterinary medical problems, leading to over 60 publications. His most recent research interests have centered on the biology of certain eye and skin tumors in cattle and horses and the localized hyperthermic treatment of eye and skin tumors and ringworm in domestic animals. Dr. Kainer taught for a year at Ross University, St. Kitts, West Indies.

Thomas O. McCracken, MS
Vice President for Product and Development
Visible Productions LLC
Fort Collins, Colorado
Mr. McCracken graduated from the University of Michigan in 1968 with a bachelor's degree in biology. He then attended graduate school at the same institution, receiving master's degrees in medical illustration, anatomy and physiology. In 1975, Mr. McCracken journeyed to Saudi Arabia where he was engaged for two years as chief medical illustrator for the King Faisal Specialist Hospital at Riyadh. Upon returning from Arabia, he accepted a position with Colorado State University as Director of Biomedical Media in the College of Veterinary Medicine and Biomedical Sciences. During the period from 1978 to 1985, he illustrated five major veterinary medical textbooks and over 75 scientific papers. In 1985, he was appointed to the faculty of the Department of Anatomy and Neurobiology, and in 1990, he became director of the sixth accredited medical illustration program in the United States, the only one associated with a veterinary medical school. Mr. McCracken resigned from CSU in 1994 to enter private enterprise, eventually assuming the vice presidency of Visible Productions. Over the years, Mr. McCracken has won numerous awards of excellence from the Association of Medical Illustrators for his anatomic and surgical illustrations. In 1997, he was the recipient of the Frank Netter Award for special contributions to medical education.

How to Use this Coloring Atlas

Using this atlas, you will explore the dog's body by coloring drawings of its various organs and reading the short descriptions accompanying the drawings. Coloring illustrations in this manner is an enjoyable and effective learning experience. In keeping with the current trend in naming parts of the body, most Latin anatomic names have been changed to English.

Drawings of **organs** making up the **systems** of the dog's body are presented in plates. Pages opposite the plates contain directions for labeling and coloring the drawings. Essential anatomic and physiologic concepts are explained and some diseases common to the region being studied are discussed. Important terms are underlined in the text.

The atlas may be used alone, or it may be used to assist in dissection. The drawings on many of the plates represent prosected specimens. For the most part, each plate is self-contained, so the plates do not have to be studied in sequence. You may select the plates you wish to color first or to review later.

Before beginning, read the following important directions:
1. Look over the entire plate on the right page, and then read instructions for labeling and coloring on the left page. The names of structures to be colored are printed in **boldface type** preceded by numbers or letters that correspond with the numbers or letters on the plate.

2. Underline the words in **boldface type** on the left page in different colors, and use the same colors on the indicated structures, arrows or dashed lines on the drawings. Also underline or color over the terms labeling structures on the drawings and color the structures where appropriate.

3. The choice of colors is yours. Colored pencils or felt-tipped pens are recommended. Suggested coloring materials include Crayola© Washable Markers, Pentel© Color Pens, colored artists' pencils, or similar media. Very dark colors obscure detail, so use lighter shades of these colors and test the colors before using them.

Surface of the Body

Regions of the Dog's Body

PLATE 1

Underline the names of the body's regions in different colors and, in matching colors, fill in the regions indicated on the drawing. You will probably have to go through your set of colors three or four times.

1. Pinna
2. Throatlatch
3. Commissure of lips
4. Flew
5. Nose
6. Muzzle
7. Foreface
8. Stop
9. Crown
10. Occiput
11. Crest
12. Neck
13. Withers
14. Shoulder

15. Point of shoulder
    (at the shoulder joint)
16. Chest
17. Arm
18. Elbow
19. Forearm
20. Carpus (wrist)
21. Metacarpus (pastern)
22. Digits (toes of the forepaw)
    1,2,3,4,5
23. Back
24. Thorax
25. Loin
26. Abdomen (belly)

27. Flank
28. Point of hip
29. Croup (rump)
30. Set of tail
31. Buttock
32. Thigh
33. Stifle (knee)
34. Leg
35. Tarsus (hock)
36. Metatarsus (pastern)
37. Dewclaw

The region called **manus** (Latin for hand) includes the carpus, metacarpus and digits.
The region called **pes** (Latin for foot) includes the tarsus, metatarsus and digits.
A **dewclaw** is a variably present first digit on the hindlimb. The term is also used to name the always present (but reduced) first digit on the forelimb.
The trunk includes all regions of the body exclusive of the head and limbs.

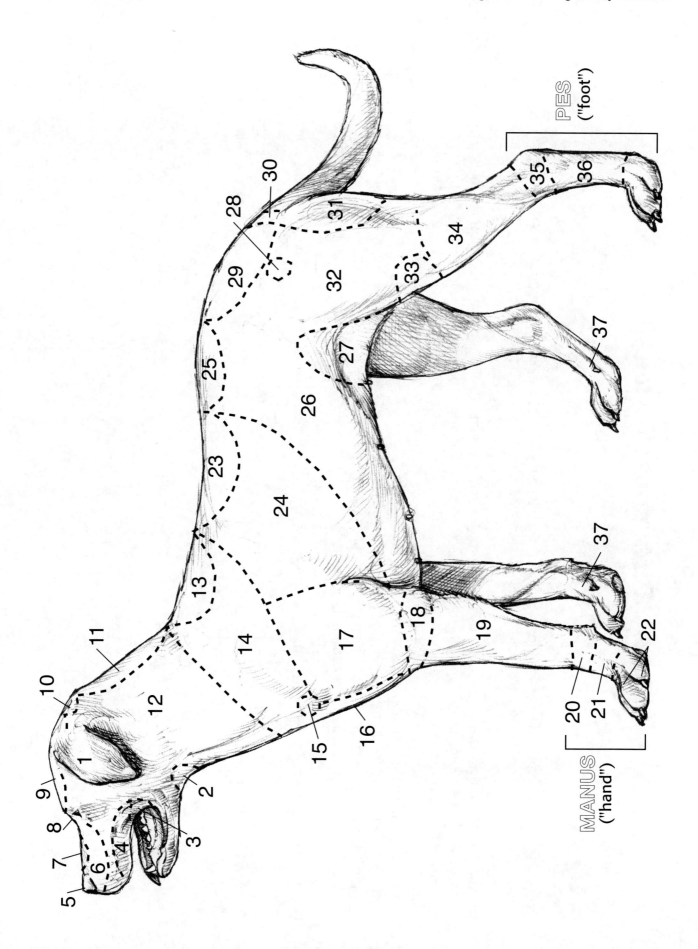

Directional Terms

PLATE 2

Directional terms (names) describe the locations of body parts, related functional changes in position, and define the extent of lesions (diseased regions). Color the words, arrows and dashed lines in matching colors.

Dorsal (A to B) and **ventral** (C to D) are opposite terms indicating the relative locations of parts toward the back, (Latin, *dorsum*) or the belly (L., *venter*).

Above the carpus (wrist) and above the tarsus (hock) and from the belly to the back, a structure located close to the cranium (skull case) is cranial to another structure. A structure located toward the tail (L., *cauda*) is **caudal** to another.

On the head, notice the dashed line from A to E. Here the anatomic term, **rostral,** is used to indicate the location of a part closer to the nose (L., rostrum). Caudal remains the same. **Proximal** indicates a location toward the attached end of a limb, that is, closer to the trunk of the body. Proximal is also used to indicate a part of the alimentary canal toward the

mouth. **Oral** is a synonym. **Distal** indicates a location toward the free end of a limb, that is, farther from the trunk. Distal is also used to indicate a part of the alimentary canal away from the mouth. **Aboral** is a synonym.

Distal to and including the carpus, **dorsal** replaces cranial and **palmar** replaces caudal. Distal to and including the tarsus, **dorsal** replaces cranial and **plantar** replaces caudal.

In reference to structures of the eye and ear, human anatomic terms are used. Anterior replaces rostral; posterior replaces caudal. On the head, superior means dorsal or upper and inferior means ventral or lower, e.g., superior palpebra means upper eyelid.

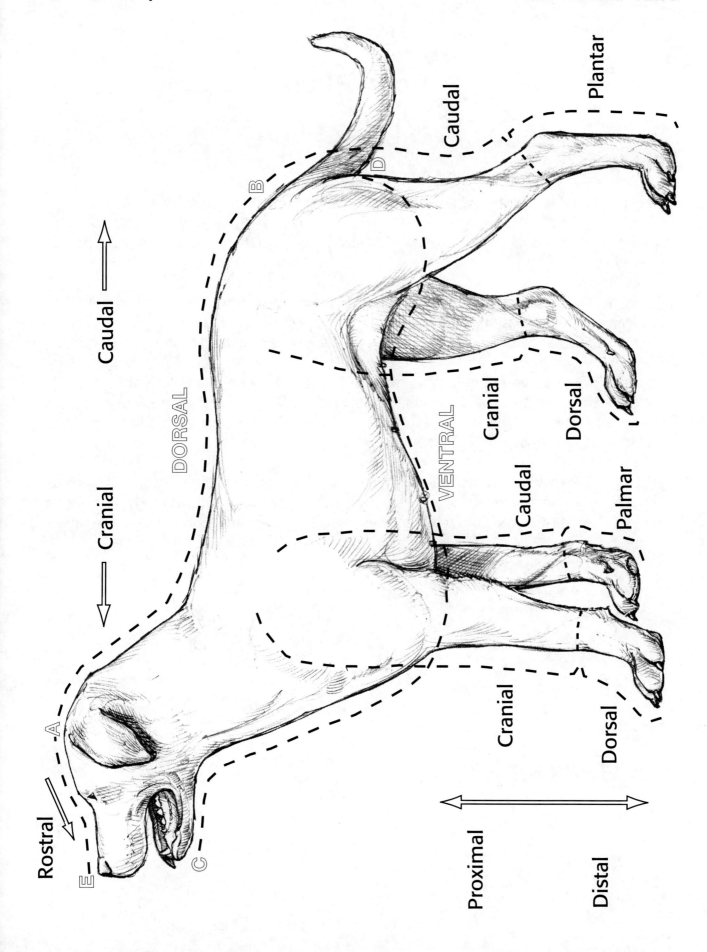

Plantar

Caudal

Cranial

Dorsal

Caudal

Palmar

Cranial

Dorsal

Caudal

DORSAL

VENTRAL

Cranial

Rostral

A

B

D

E

C

Proximal

Distal

Body Planes

PLATE 3

Body planes are formed by any two points that can be connected by a straight line.

Filll in words, arrows, and dashed lines in different colors. Color the four body plane panels very lightly.

Figure 1. The **median plane** (L., *medianus* = in the middle), indicated by dashed lines between the m's, divides the dog's body into right and left halves. A **sagittal plane** (L., *sagitta* = arrow), indicated by the dashed line from s to s, is any plane parallel to the median plane.

Figure 2. The **median plane** is indicated by a dashed line. **Medial** and **lateral** (L., *latus* = flank) are directional terms relative to the median plane. Medial structures are "inside", located closer to the median plane. Lateral structures are "outside", away from the median plane, that is, toward the flank or side.

Figure 3. A **transverse plane**, indicated by a dashed line between the t's, passes through the head, trunk or limb perpendicular to the long axis of the part. A **dorsal plane (frontal plane)**, indicated by a dashed line from d to d, passes through a body part parallel to its dorsal surface.

Figure 1

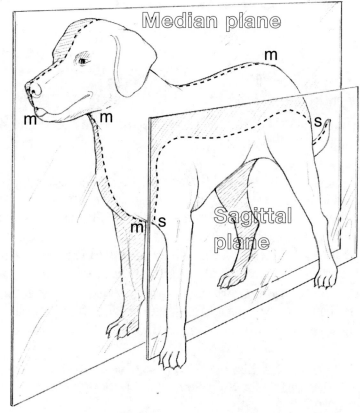

Figure 2

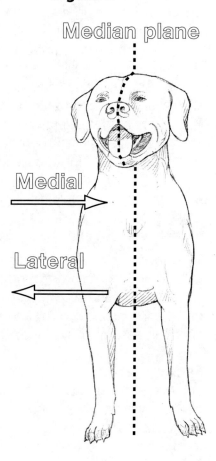

Figure 3

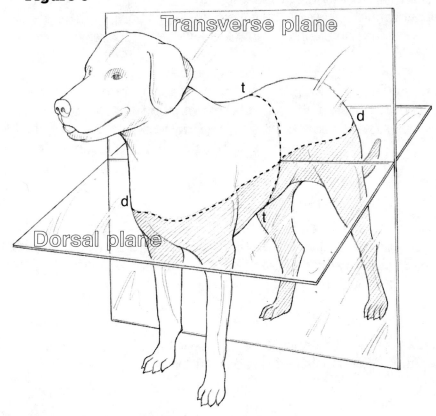

Anatomy of Canine Skin

PLATE 4

Figure 1. Low power microscopic view of a block of haired skin from the flank. Using different colors, color names and structures indicated.

Skin consists of **epidermis** and **dermis**, the latter blending into a **hypodermis (subcutis)** that attaches the dermis to underlying structures and protects the skin from excessive pressures.

Epidermis is stratified squamous epithelium, a many-celled tissue with horny, flat, overlapping surface cells. This tissue continues down into the dermis, forming hair follicles containing the hair roots. The **hair bulb matrix** at the end of each follicle is in contact with a nourishing, vessel-rich **dermal papilla**. Cells in the hair bulb matrix multiply to form the hair. Canine skin has **compound follicles** consisting of a **primary follicle** producing a large **guard (cover) hair** and several smaller **secondary follicles** producing the fine **wool (vellus) hairs** of the undercoat. Both types of hair emerge on the surface through the same pore. The outer surface of a hair is formed by overlapping, cornified scales. The deep layers of the epidermis and the hair bulb matrix produce pigment. Make dots with a black pencil to indicate **pigment cells.**

Dermis is dense fibrous (collagenous) connective tissue, and the **subcutis** is loose connective tissue containing masses of fat cells (adipose tissue). Both tissues contain blood vessels, nerves, white blood cells and other cells of the immune system.

Two types of glands empty into hair follicles. Cells produced by oil (**sebaceous**) **glands** break up to form the oily secretion, sebum. Coiled tubular **sweat (apocrine) glands** secrete a thick, "dry" sweat. Sweat and sebum move out on the hairs. An oval to elongated tail gland area on the dorsum of the tail contains large oil and sweat gands. Single hair shafts here are large and stiff. There are no glands in nasal skin. Moisture on the surface here comes from glands in the nasal cavity.

Sensory nerves bring sensations of pressure, tension, pain, itching, heat and cold from nerve endings in the dermis. **Motor nerves** (from the sympathetic nervous system) cause the apocrine glands to secrete sweat and smooth muscle cells of the **hair erector muscles** to contract. Contractions of these muscles elevate hairs and squeeze oil glands. **Blood vessels** branch and join to form three networks in the subcutis and dermis. Lymph capillary networks begin around hair follicles and skin glands.

Figure 2. Microscopic view of a tactile hair from the muzzle.

A very sensitive **tactile (sinus) hair**, such as a large, dark hair on the muzzle or over the eyes, is a single hair with its follicle surrounded by a connective tissue sheath containing blood-fllled **venous sinuses**. The endings of numerous **sensory nerves** in the connective tissue sheath pick up slight movements of the tactile hair increased through hydraulic pressure by the blood in the sinuses.

Figure 3. Microscopic view of nonhaired skin from a footpad.

Tubular **merocrine glands** in the fatty tissue of the digital cushion deliver a watery secretion through passages in the thick epidermis of the nonhaired skin of the footpad.

Figure 1

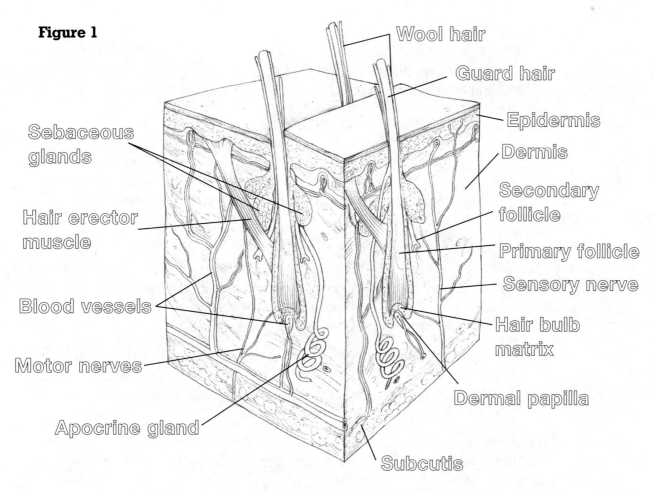

Wool hair

Guard hair

Epidermis

Dermis

Secondary follicle

Primary follicle

Sensory nerve

Hair bulb matrix

Dermal papilla

Subcutis

Sebaceous glands

Hair erector muscle

Blood vessels

Motor nerves

Apocrine gland

Figure 2

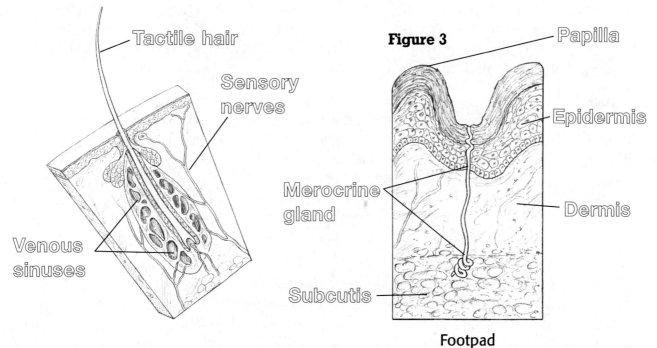

Tactile hair

Sensory nerves

Venous sinuses

Figure 3

Papilla

Epidermis

Dermis

Merocrine gland

Subcutis

Footpad

Functions of Canine Skin

PLATE 5

The skin is the largest organ in the body - 11%-25% of body weight, being highest in puppies. As a <u>sensory organ</u>, its nerve endings provide information to the central nervous system on pressure, tension, pain, itching, and temperature. Color names and structures indicated.

Figure 1. Section (slice) of canine skin. Higher magnification.
<u>Keratinocytes</u> (cells of the epidermis) multiply in the **basal layer** of the tissue. They change shape, becoming flat and <u>cornified</u> (<u>horny</u>) as they are moved to the **cornified layer (stratum corneum)** where they die. This process takes about three weeks. The cornified, flat, dead cells remain in the layers of the stratum corneum for another three weeks before they are shed. Millions of surface cells are shed each day.

In contact with the environment, the skin serves as a <u>barrier</u> to intrusion by living things (viruses, bacteria and larger parasites) and by physical and chemical agents. Protection is afforded by the cornified, dead, surface cells of the epidermis and by white blood cells and other immune system cells in the dermis. Water resistance is furnished by the surface cells of the epidermis, the dense hairs of the undercoat, and the oily sebum produced by the sebaceous glands.

The skin lends <u>flexible support</u> to underlying structures, and the subcutis lets the skin glide over them. This arrangement permits the skin to be shaken from side to side and recoil (as when shaking off water) without the dog losing balance. When a dog is dehydrated, the skin does not snap back quickly when it is pinched and released.

<u>Regulation of body temperature</u> is aided by the skin. Blood vessels in the dermis and subcutis contract to reduce blood volume near the surface, thus conserving body heat. In a hot environment, blood vessels expand, bringing more blood near the surface to give off heat. The dog's apocrine tubular (sweat) glands produce only a scant, thick secretion that does not wet the skin as does the sweat of horses and people. In dogs, cooling the body is helped by <u>panting</u>. With the mouth open, air flowing back and forth over the tongue tends to cool blood in its superficial vessels. <u>Blood pressure control</u> is assisted through contraction and expansion of blood vessels in the dermis and subcutis.

Figure 2. Hair cycle.
<u>Production of hair</u> is a joint task between a **dermal papilla** and a **hair bulb matrix**. The hair cycle includes an actively growing stage (**anagen**) followed by a stage (**catagen**) during which the hair bulb matrix sort of shrinks and peels away from its blood supply in the dermal papilla. A longer, quiescent period (**telogen**) then takes place. The hair (now a **club hair**) separates from the hair bulb matrix but remains in the follicle. The hair bulb matrix later becomes active, contacts the dermal papilla and begins to grow a new hair. The new, growing hair pushes out the old club hair (<u>shedding</u>). Hairs are shed periodically, mostly in the spring, but, in some breeds, shedding may occur throughout the year.

Diseases such as hypothyroidism (decreased production of thyroid hormones) and Cushing's disease (increased production of hormones by the adrenal cortex) can contribute to skin problems. <u>Alopecia</u> (loss of hair), reddening and crusting of the skin, and generalized demodectic mange are all accompanied by <u>pruritis</u> (itching) and may be manifestations of systemic disease.

Figure 1

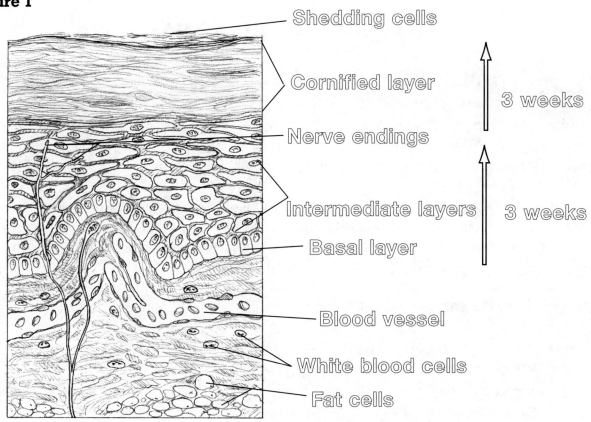

Shedding cells

Cornified layer

3 weeks

Nerve endings

Intermediate layers   3 weeks

Basal layer

Blood vessel

White blood cells

Fat cells

Figure 2

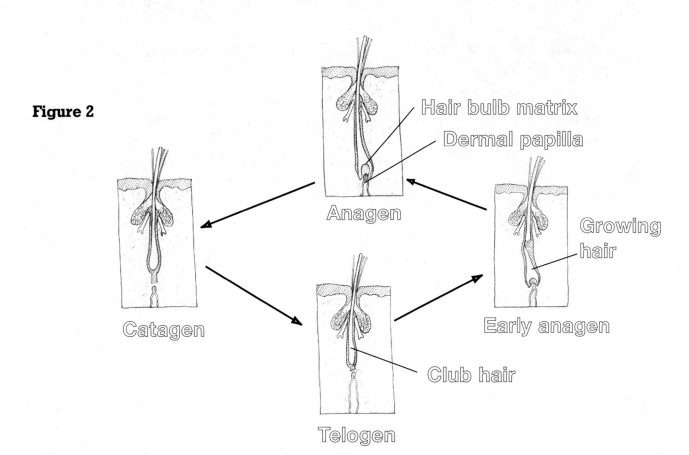

Hair bulb matrix

Dermal papilla

Anagen

Growing hair

Catagen

Early anagen

Club hair

Telogen

Types of Hair Coats

PLATE 6

Dog hairs vary from straight or bristly guard hairs to the wavy wool hairs of the undercoat and the softest wool hairs (vellus hairs) of puppies. Vellus hairs are the puppy's only hairs in the first few weeks after birth. Then the guard hairs emerge from their follicles.

Adult dogs of most breeds possess a **double coat**. Guard hairs form a protective, outer **cover coat**; finer wool hairs make up the **undercoat**. The undercoat supports the cover coat, providing an insulating, water-resistant barrier. Longer guard hairs form the feathering on limbs, the plumes on tails and the ruff around the neck in certain breeds.

The typical **double coat** is seen in the Siberian Husky, German Shepherd, several terrier breeds and in the majority of crossbred dogs.
Variations of the double coat include:

The **corded coat** of dogs such as the Komondor and Puli.

The **long coat** of the Poodle. Contrary to the popular belief that Poodles have a single coat, this breed possesses a double coat and sheds hairs. The Poodle's cover coat of thick, close curls forms cords if left to grow uncombed and unclipped. Overall, the coat lends itself to the different Poodle clips.

The **broken (wiry) coat** of harsh, wiry guard hairs and a soft undercoat of the Wire Fox Terrier. The hairs of this breed are often plucked (or "stripped").

The **medium coat** of spaniels and setters with wavy guard hairs over the undercoat.

The **curly coat** of certain sporting dogs (Curly-coated Retriever, Irish Water Spaniel) is a mass of crisp curls.

A **single** coat lacks an undercoat. The uniform hairs may be short as on Pointers and Italian Greyhounds or long as on the toy breeds Papillon and Maltese.

The skin of a hairless dog contains a few stunted hairs. Larger hairs appear on the head (crest), tail (plume), manus and pes (socks). The skin of these dogs contains well-developed, active sweat glands.

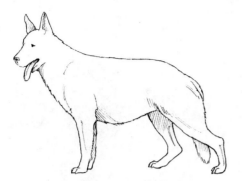

Double coat

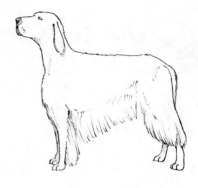

Medium coat

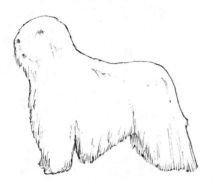

Corded coat

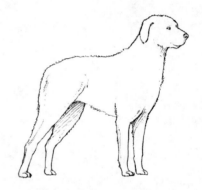

Curly coat

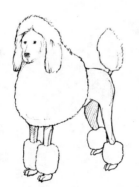

Long coat

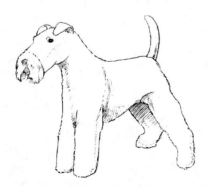

Broken coat

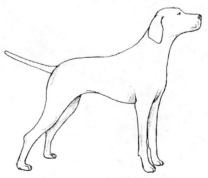

Single coat

Organs of Movement:
Bones, Joints, and Muscles

Skeleton of the Dog

PLATE 7

There are around 320 bones in the dog's body, including 3 <u>ossicles</u> (little bones) in each temporal bone of the skull. The tiny clavicle is located in the clavicular tendon of the brachiocephalic muscle.

Underline the name of each bone with a different color and use the same color on the labeled bone.

AXIAL SKELETON

1. Skull
2. Mandible
3. Hyoid apparatus
4. Vertebral column
5. Ribs
6. Costal cartilages
7. Sternum
30. Penile bone (baculum)

APPENDICULAR SKELETON

8. Clavicle
9. Scapula
10. Humerus
11. Radius
12. Ulna

FORELIMB

13. Carpal bones (7)
14. Metacarpal bones (5)
15. Palmar sesamoid bones (9)
16. Proximal phalanges (5)
17. Middle phalanges (4)
18. Dorsal sesamoid bones (4)
19. Distal phalanges (5)
    (Singular = phalanx)

HINDLIMB

20. Ilium ⎫
21. Pubis ⎬ Fused to form the hip bone
22. Ischium ⎭ (es coxae)
23. Femur
24. Patella
25. Fabellae (3)
26. Tibia
27. Fibula
28. Tarsal bones (7)
29. Metatarsal bones (5)

Hindlimb digital bones are named the same as those of the forelimb. A dewclaw (1st digit) is rarely present.

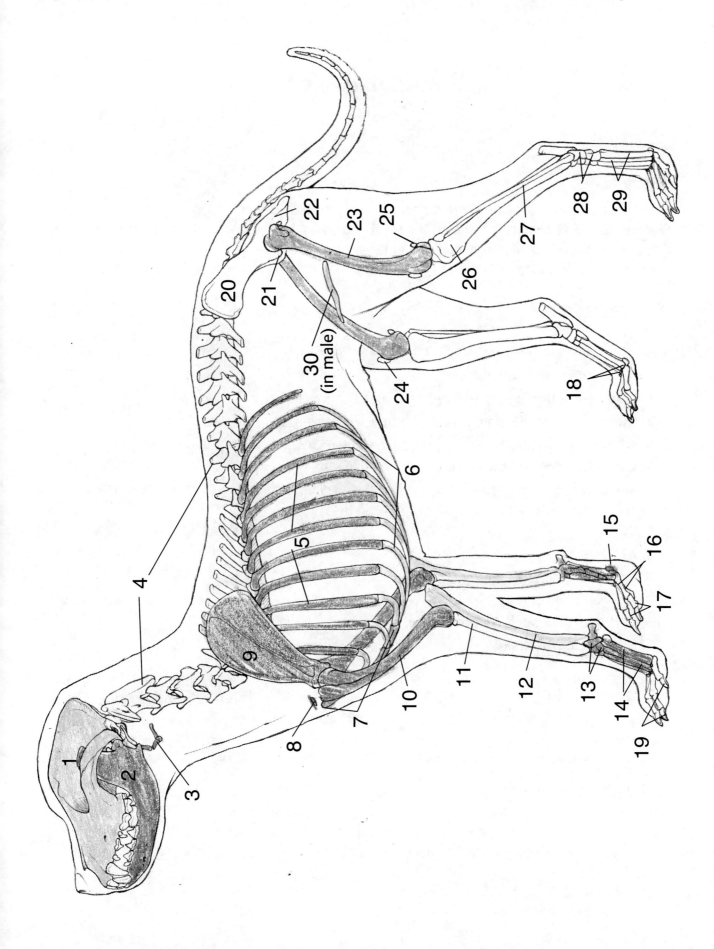

Vertebral Column

PLATE 8

Figure 1. Regions of the vertebral (spinal) column.

Color in the vertebral regions and the number of vertebrae in each region:
7 cervical, 13 thoracic, 7 lumbar, 3 sacral (fused by 1 1/2 years to form the **sacrum**) and **20** (more or less) **caudal (coccygeal) vertebrae.**
Next to the wide variation in the number of caudal vertebrae, the most common variation is 6 lumbar vertebrae.
The vertebral formula of the dog is written $C_7 \, T_{13} \, L_7 \, S_3 \, Ca_{20}$.

Figure 2. Vertebrae are irregular bones of various shapes.

Identify and color the parts of vertebrae from different regions:
1. **Transverse processes** (**Wings** on the atlas and sacrum)
2. **Dens** of the axis (Held down by the transverse ligament of the atlas)
3. **Transverse foramen** (On all cervical vertebrae except the seventh)
4. **Lateral vertebral foramen**
5. **Vertebral foramen** (Combined vertebral foramina form the vertebral canal which contains and protects the spinal cord and its coverings.)
6. **Body**
7. **Arch**
8. **Spinous process(es)**
9. **Articular processes**
10. **Left articular surface of sacrum**. (Articulates with ilium)
11. **Intervertebral disks**

Except for articulations of the atlas with the skull (atlanto-occipital joint) and with the axis (atlanto-axial joint - a pivot joint), the bodies of vertebrae are joined by **intervertebral disks** of fibrocartilage. These discs are relatively thick in the dog, accounting for one sixth of the length of the vertebral column. Movements of vertebral joints (except the atlanto-axial joint) are dorsal, ventral and lateral flexion. There is also limited rotation.

Spinal nerves come out through foramina formed between arches of adjacent vertebrae or through lateral vertebral foramina in arches. On each side, a vertebral artery runs through foramina in the transverse processes of cervical vertebrae six through one (the atlas) and through the lateral vertebral foramen of the atlas to contribute to the blood supply to the brain.

Figure 1

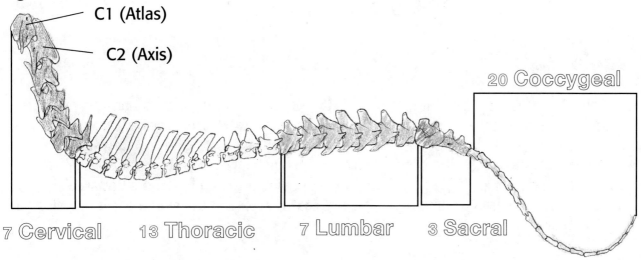

C1 (Atlas)

C2 (Axis)

20 Coccygeal

7 Cervical   13 Thoracic   7 Lumbar   3 Sacral

Figure 2

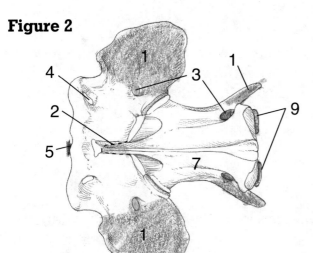

Atlas and Axis

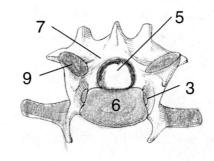

Cervical vertebra IV

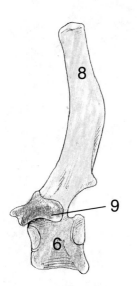

Thoracic vertebra

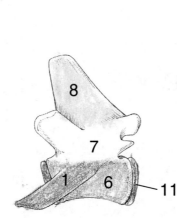

Lumbar vertebra

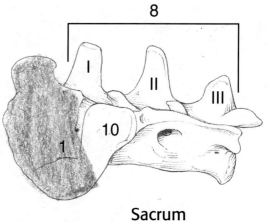

Sacrum

Ribs and Sternum

PLATE 9

The dog has 13 pairs (rarely 12 or 14 pairs) of **ribs** (L., *costa* = rib), each rib consisting of a bony part joined to a **costal cartilage** at a **costochondral junction** (Greek, *chondros* = cartilage). The costal cartilages of the first nine pairs of ribs articulate with the **sternum** at **chondrosternal junctions**; the last four pairs are asternal ribs. Since their cartilages do not attach to adjacent costal cartilages, the **13th ribs** are called floating ribs. Fused costal cartilages form the **costal arch**. Most of the bony ribs, the **costal arch** and the sternum can be palpated (felt) from the exterior.

Figure 1. Left lateral view of ribs, sternum and vertebrae.

The **head** of each rib one through 10 or 11 articulates with the bodies of adjacent vertebrae and the intervertebral disc between them. The head of the **first rib** articulates with the bodies of the **7th cervical (C7)** and **1st thoracic (T1) vertebrae**. Ribs 11 or 12 through 13 articulate only with thoracic vertebrae of the same number. The **tubercle** on ribs one through 10 or 11 articulates with the transverse process of the thoracic vertebra of the same number. On the caudal ribs of the series, the **neck** of the rib becomes shorter as the tubercle approaches the head and eventually fuses with it.

Figure 2. Ventral view of ribs and sternum.

The **sternum** consists of eight elongated, bony **sternebrae** joined by **intersternal cartilages**. The first sternebra is called the **manubrium**; the eighth sternebra, the **xiphoid process**. A thin, flat plate, the **xiphoid cartilage**, extends caudad from the xiphoid process.

Figure 1

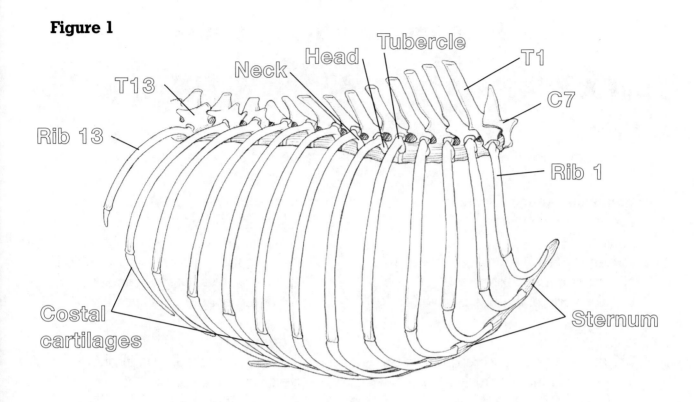

Figure 2

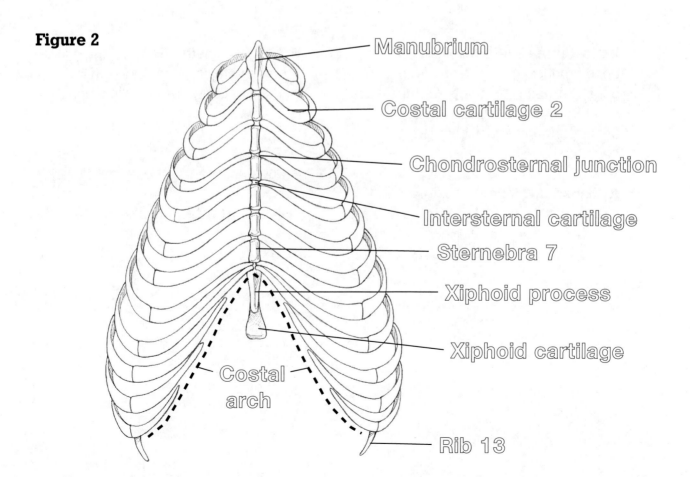

Anatomy of a Long Bone

PLATE 10

Longitudinal section of a mature canine humerus.

Color the names and the regions indicated on the drawing. Coloring suggested below.

1. **Diaphysis (shaft)** - Arrow indicates extent. Color the arrow.

2. **Epiphysis (end)** - Arrows indicate an epiphysis at the proximal end and one at the distal end of the bone. Color the arrows.

3. **Epiphyseal line** - Each epiphyseal line is the region of the final replacement of growth plate cartilage by bone (see Plate 11).

4. **Periosteum** - This is the vessel-rich, bone-producing membrane covering the bone (dashed line) except over the ends covered by articular cartilage. Color periosteum and endosteum (9. below) black.

5. **Articular cartilage** - Smooth, hyaline (glassy) cartilage covers the ends of a bone where it meets another bone in a joint. Color the cartilage blue.

6. **Cancellous (spongy) bone** - Bony trabeculae (little beams) give support against stresses placed on a bone. Red bone marrow (source of most blood cells) occupies spaces among trabeculae. Color red bone marrow red.

7. **Compact bone** - This tissue is formed by densely-packed, cylindrical osteons of cells and bone matrix containing channels for blood vessels. Color compact bone brown.

8. **Marrow cavity** - Fatty yellow bone marrow replaces red bone marrow in the marrow cavity. Color yellow bone marrow yellow.

9. **Endosteum** - Bone is laid down by this membrane lining the marrow cavity.

10. **Nutrient artery** - Blood for the bone is supplied by vessels in the periosteum and by the nutrient artery carrying blood to the endosteum. Color nutrient artery red.

Long bone
(Humerus)

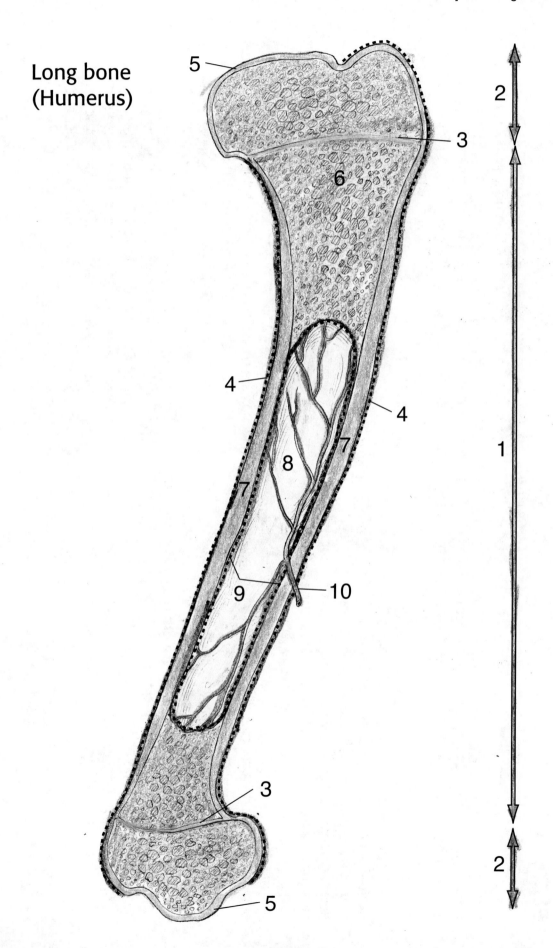

Bone Development

PLATE 11

Most bones develop in a mass of cartilage (endochondral ossification) in the fetus (unborn). Some bones of the skull develop in membranes of collagenous connective tissue (intramembranous ossification); in others, both types of bone formation occur.

Blood vessels and bone-forming cells from developing **periosteum** invade a **cartilage model** of a bone to establish a **primary center of ossification**. Bone-forming cells lay down temporary bone on calcified cartilage. Much remodeling takes place through the activity of bone-destroying and bone-forming cells as the cartilage model is replaced by bone. A **marrow cavity** is hollowed out. Compact bone around the outside and supporting spongy bone are finally formed.

Secondary centers of ossification are formed at each **epiphysis** of a long bone. Cartilage between the primary and secondary centers of ossification, the **growth plate (physis)**, continues to grow and is changed to bone during puppy-hood, causing the bone to grow in length. Peripheral growth is provided by bone-forming cells in the periosteum, except where **articular cartilage** remains, and in the endosteum.

On the following diagrams, suggested colors are blue for cartilage, light brown for bone and red for blood vessels.

Figure 1. Cartilage model of a long bone with a primary center of ossification.
Figure 2. Secondary centers of ossification in the two epiphyses of a developing long bone.
Figure 3. Developing long bone after birth with active growth plates.

Achondroplasia is a genetic (inherited) defect that limits the growth of cartilage. Restricted growth of cartilage results in a form of dwarfism primarily involving the long limb bones of young, growing dogs. Recall that the growth of a long bone depends on the conversion of proliferating growth plate cartilage to bone. While the head and trunk develop normally, the limbs are short, stunted and often bowed. The limb bones, however, are as strong as normal bones. This is standard conformation of Dachshunds, Bassett Hounds and English Bulldogs.

Achondroplasia can also occur in the axial skeleton where it is seen in the screw tail of the Boston Terrier and the extreme shortening of the head in this breed, the Pekingese and the English Bulldog. Overshot and undershot jaws are caused by abnormal intramembranous development of upper and lower jaws.

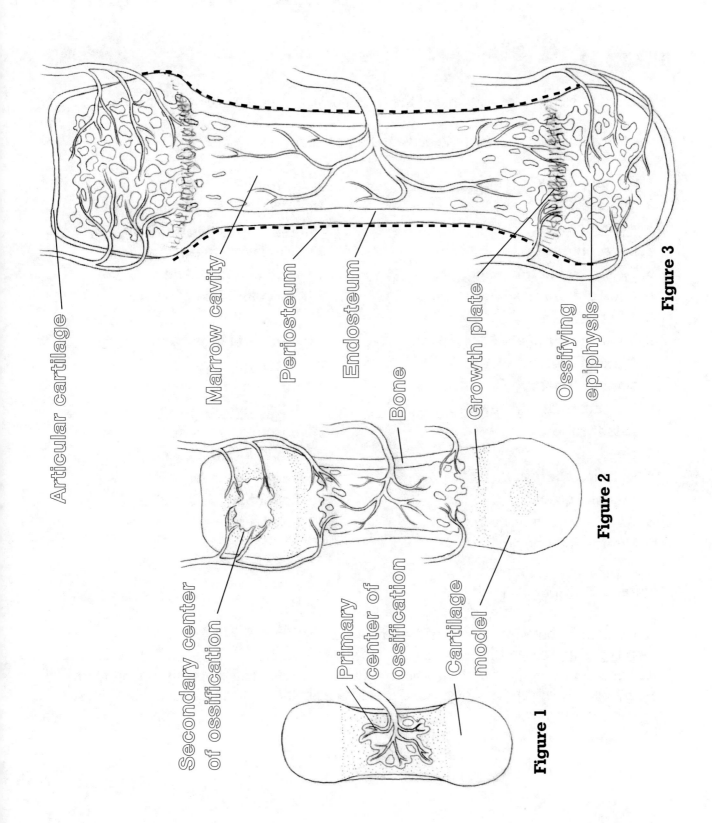

Articular cartilage

Marrow cavity

Periosteum

Endosteum

Bone

Growth plate

Ossifying
epiphysis

Secondary center
of ossification

Primary
center of
ossification

Cartilage
model

Figure 3

Figure 2

Figure 1

Bones of the Shoulder, Arm, and Forearm

PLATE 12

Figure 1. Lateral and medial views of the left scapula, humerus, radius and ulna.

Underline the names and color the parts of the bones different colors.

1. Supraspinous fossa
2. Spine
3. Acromion
4. Infraspinous fossa
5. Supraglenoid tubercle
6. Coracoid process
7. Serrated face
8. Subscapular fossa
9. Glenoid cavity
10. Greater tubercle
11. Intertubercular groove
12. Lesser tubercle
13. Head
14. Deltoid tuberosity
15. Brachial groove
16. Teres major tuberosity
17. Lateral epicondyle

18. Capitulum
19. Trochlea
20. Supratrochlear foramen
21. Olecranon fossa
22. Medial epicondyle
23. Articular circumference
24. Neck
25. Radial tuberosity
26. Olecranon process
27. Coronoid process
    – lateral projection
28. Coronoid process
    – medial projection
29. Carpal articular surface
30. Styloid process – ulna
31. Styloid process – radius

Figure 2. Skeleton of a Dachshund.

Short, deformed but strong bones of the limbs of a Dachshund are the result of hereditary achondroplasia, a congenital disturbance in growth and maturation of epiphyseal cartilage, causing inadequate endochondral formation of bone. Lack of sufficient limb support for the long, heavy trunk of this breed and degenerative processes in the centers of intervertebral discs lead to protrusion of the intervertebral discs ("slipped discs"), particularly in the lumbar region. Slipped discs place pressure upon spinal nerve roots.

Figure 1

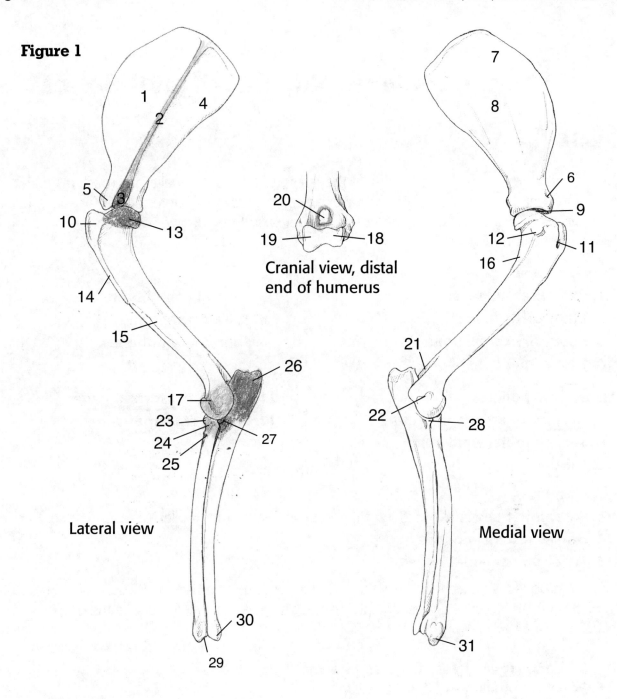

Cranial view, distal
end of humerus

Lateral view

Medial view

Figure 2

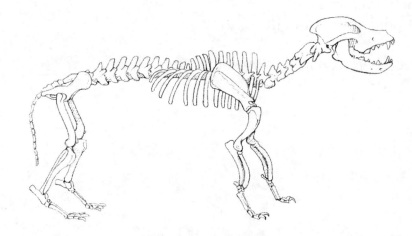

Carpal, Metacarpal, and Digital Bones

PLATE 13

Dorsal and palmar views of the bones of the left carpus (wrist), metacarpus (pastern) and forefoot (forepaw) with the bones slightly disarticulated. Using a different color for each of the four groups below, underline the names of the bones in the group. Use the same colors for the labeled bones on the plate.

Carpal bones:
1. Radial carpal bone
2. Ulnar carpal bone
3. Accessory carpal bone
4. First carpal bone

5. Second carpal bone
6. Third carpal bone
7. Fourth carpal bone

Metacarpal bones:
8. First metacarpal bone
9. Second metacarpal bone
10. Third metacarpal bone

11. Fourth metacarpal bone
12. Fifth metacarpal bone

Sesamoid bones:
13. **Sesamoid bone** in the tendon of the long abductor of the pollex (thumb).
14. **Dorsal sesamoid bones**
15. **Proximal sesamoid bones**

Sesamoid bones are attached to or embedded in tendons of muscles. A sesamoid bone protects a tendon where it moves against a joint surface, acting as a pulley to change the tendon's direction of pull.

Digital bones (phalanges; singular, phalanx):
16. Proximal phalanges - I, II, III, IV, V
17. Middle phalanges - II, III, IV, V
18. Distal phalanges - I, II, III, IV, V

On each distal phalanx note the **ungual crest** and **ungual process** which is enclosed by the claw.

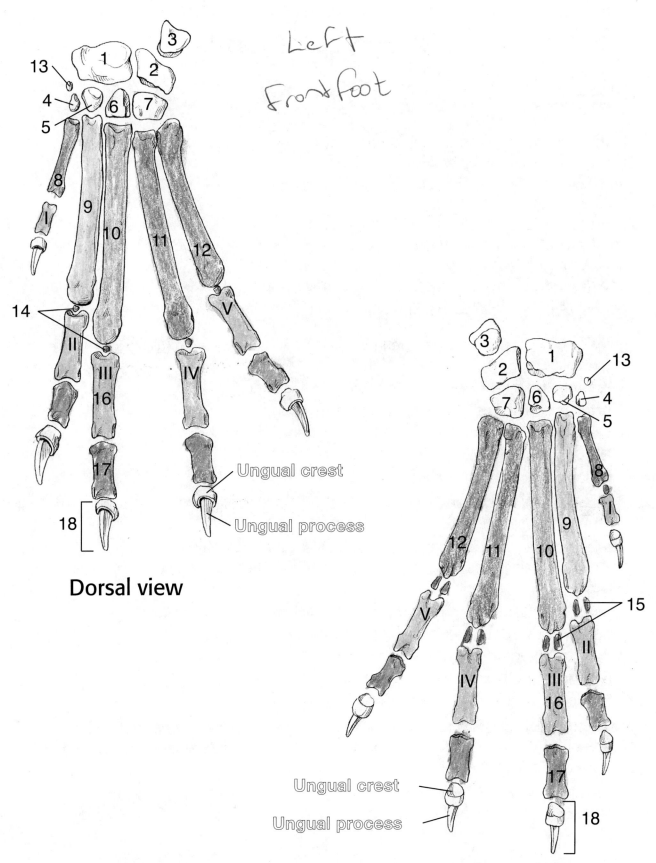

Left
Front foot

Dorsal view

Ungual crest

Ungual process

Palmar view

Ungual crest

Ungual process

Structure of Joints

PLATE 14

Figure 1. Fibrous joints - Immovable; united by fibrous tissue; ossify with age.
Suture - Most joints of the skull.
Syndesmosis - Between the shafts of some long bones.

Figure 2. Cartilaginous joints - Limited movement; midline.
Symphysis - Fibrocartilage. Pelvic symphysis ossifies with age. Intervertebral discs do not normally ossify.
Growth plate (physis) (arrows) - Hyaline cartilage grows and ossifies (changes to bone), increasing a bone's length. It completely ossifies at maturity.

Figure 3. Synovial joint - Drawn here in longitudinal section. Synovial (diarthrodial) joints are movable.

Parts of a typical synovial joint. Color the parts indicated.
Articular cartilages - Smooth, glassy hyaline cartilage.
Synovial membrane - Produces lubricating synovial fluid ("joint oil").
Fibrous joint capsule
Collateral ligaments - Extra-articular.
Intra-articular ligaments in the femorotibial joint of the stifle (knee) are not within the synovial cavity. In this joint, menisci of fibrocartilage are placed between the articulating bones.

Synovial joints are classified also on the basis of the shape of articular surfaces and type of motion:
Hinge joint (ginglymus) - Flexion decreases the angle between the bones in a joint; extension increases the angle: elbow joint.
Sliding joint (plane joint): intercarpal joints - between carpal bones.
Ball-and-socket joint (spheroidal joint): hip joint.
Pivot joint (trochoid joint): atlanto-axial joint.
Ellipsoid joint - Biaxial movement: antebrachiocarpal joint.
Saddle joints : the dog's interphalangeal joints.

The initial swelling of an injured joint is due to increased production of synovial fluid. Analysis of the viscosity (thickness) of the synovial fluid and cells that it contains is used to diagnose certain joint diseases.

Growth plate fractures occur in very young dogs before the growth plate ossifies.

Figure 1. Fibrous joints

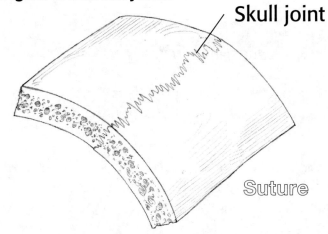

Skull joint

Suture

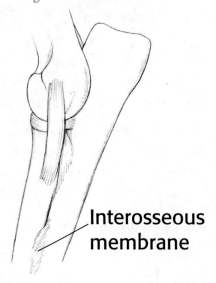

Syndesmosis

Interosseous membrane

Figure 2. Cartilaginous joints

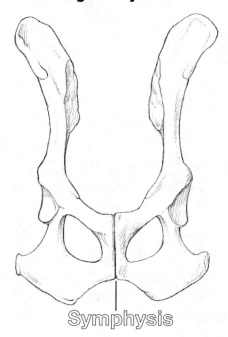

Symphysis

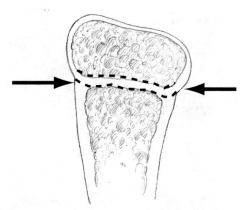

Growth plate (physis)

Figure 3. Synovial joint

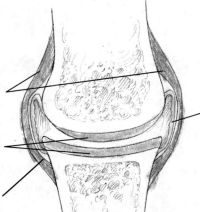

Collateral ligaments

Articular cartilage

Fibrous joint capsule

Synovial membrane

Joints of the Forelimb

PLATE 15

On the plate, color the names and draw a colored line through the joints indicated.

Shoulder (humeral) joint - Glenoid cavity of scapula with head of humerus. Surrounding muscles act as ligaments. This is a ball-and-socket joint but main movements are flexion and extension.

Elbow (cubital) joint - Condyle of humerus with capitular fovea of radius and trochlear notch of ulna. It includes the **proximal radioulnar joint** between the articular circumference of the radius and the radial notch of the ulna. The joint capsule extends a pouch into the olecranon fossa. The elbow joint is a ginglymus with some rotation.

Interosseous ligament of the antebrachium - Between apposed rough areas on the shafts of the radius and ulna.

Distal radioulnar joint - Between radius and ulna distally. Contains an extension of the antebrachiocarpal joint capsule. Allows some rotation.

Carpal joints - Together act as a ginglymus.
   Antebrachiocarpal joint - Between distal ends of radius and ulna and proximal row of carpal bones. Major joint of the carpus.
   Midddle carpal joint - Between proximal row and distal row of carpal bones.
   Carpometacarpal joint - Between distal row of carpal bones and proximal ends (bases) of metacarpal bones.
   Intercarpal joints - Between individual carpal bones.

Several small ligaments between adjacent bones, short radial carpal ligaments and a short ulnar carpal ligament bind the carpal joints. The palmar carpal fibrocartilage attaches to all of the carpal bones except the accessory carpal and forms the deep smooth surface of the carpal canal. The fibrous flexor retinaculum and accessory carpal bone complete the formation of the canal, enclosing digital flexor tendons, blood vessels, and nerves.

Intermetacarpal joints - Between proximal ends of adjacent metacarpal bones.

Metacarpophalangeal joints - Between distal ends of metacarpal bones and proximal ends of proximal phalanges. Various sesamoidean ligaments stabilize the pair of palmar sesamoid bones embedded in the tendon of the interosseous muscle at each of the four main joints.

Proximal interphalangeal joints - Between proximal and middle phalanges.

Distal interphalangeal joints - Between middle and distal phalanges. Collateral ligaments bind the interphalangeal joints. A dorsal elastic ligament extends from the middle phalanx to the ungual crest of the distal phalanx.

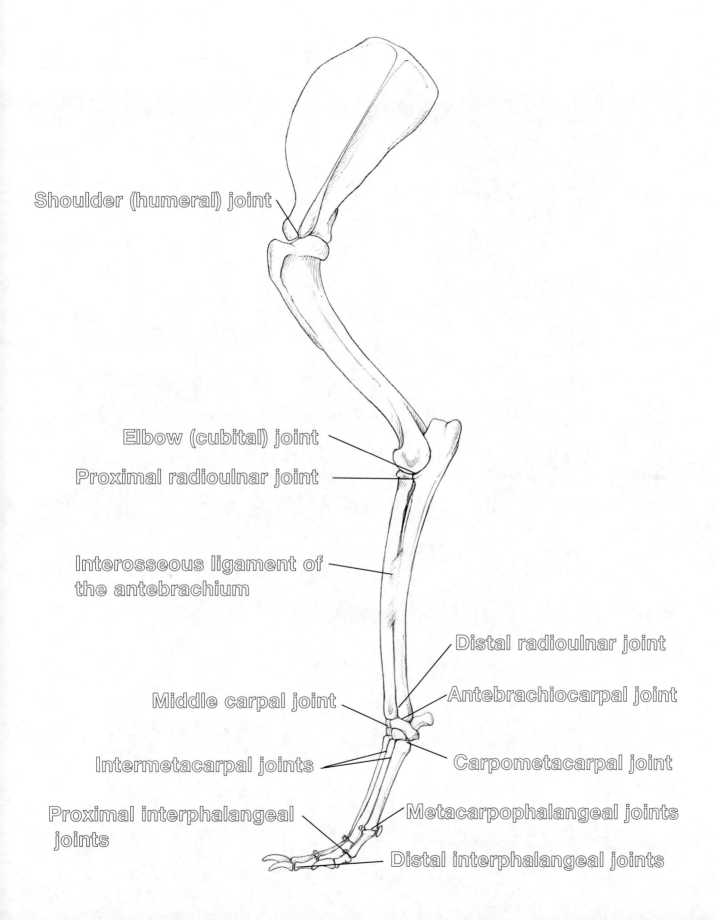

Shoulder (humeral) joint

Elbow (cubital) joint

Proximal radioulnar joint

Interosseous ligament of
the antebrachium

Distal radioulnar joint

Antebrachiocarpal joint

Middle carpal joint

Intermetacarpal joints

Carpometacarpal joint

Proximal interphalangeal
joints

Metacarpophalangeal joints

Distal interphalangeal joints

Fascia

PLATE 16

When removing the skin from an animal, the lacy subcutis of loose connective tissue is seen as it is pulled away from the superficial fascia. The latter varies from loose to dense connective tissue that envelops the body and contains certain cutaneous muscles of the head, neck and trunk. The largest of these is the m. cutaneus trunci (cutaneous muscle of the trunk) that covers a large part of the thorax and abdomen. Deep to the superficial fascia, thick, white deep fascia of heavier, dense connective tissue encloses muscles and sends partitions called septa between muscles and some muscle parts. Before the limits of many muscles can be seen clearly, fascia has to be cleaned, that is, removed. Fascia covers joints and blends with ligaments, tendons and tendon sheaths.

Color the names of the region of fascia (large dashed line) and the cutaneous muscles. Color the cutaneous muscles (small dashed line).

MAJOR REGIONS OF FASCIA
Fascia of the head
Cervical fascia
Omobrachial fascia
Spinotransverse fascia
  (deep to the shoulder)
Thoracolumbar fascia
Abdominal fascia
Gluteal fascia
Tail fascia
Lateral femoral fascia (Fascia lata)
Medial femoral fascia
  (on medial aspect of the thigh)
Crural fascia

CUTANEOUS MUSCLES
Platysma muscle
Sphincter muscles of the neck
Cutaneous muscle of the trunk (m. cutaneus trunci)

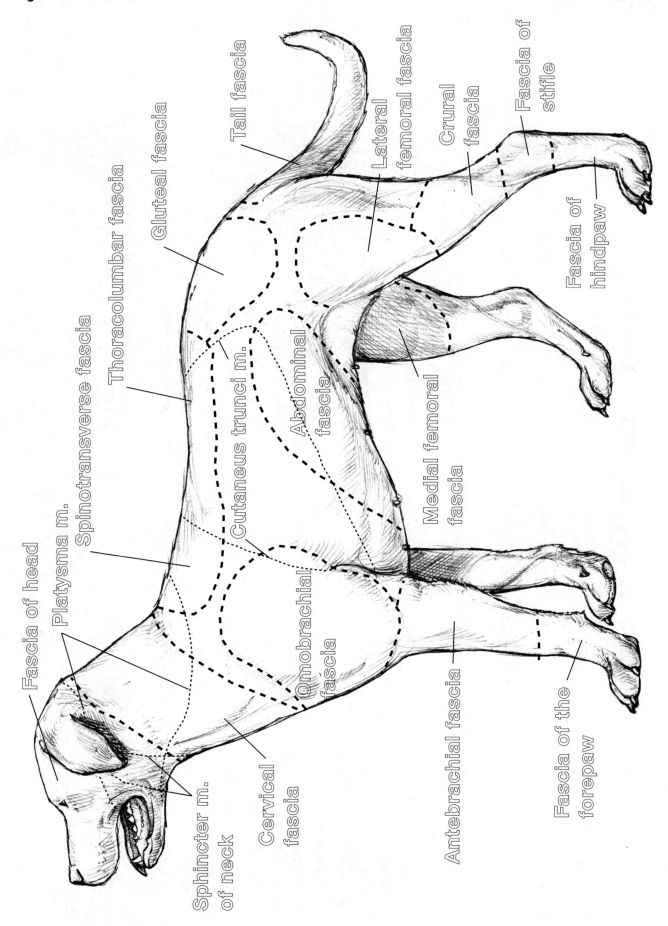

Fascia of head

Platysma m.

Spinotransverse fascia

Thoracolumbar fascia

Gluteal fascia

Tail fascia

Lateral femoral fascia

Crural fascia

Fascia of stifle

Fascia of hindpaw

Medial femoral fascia

Abdominal fascia

Cutaneus trunci m.

Omobrachial fascia

Sphincter m. of neck

Cervical fascia

Antebrachial fascia

Fascia of the forepaw

Superficial Muscles of the Dog

PLATE 17

Left lateral view of the superficial muscles after removal of most of the fascia and the cutaneous muscles.

Underline names and color the muscles indicated on the drawing. m. = muscle. The cleidocervical m. and cleidobrachial m. are parts of the brachiocephalic m.

1. Nasolabial levator m.
2. Orbicular ocular m.
3. Zygomatic m.
4. Frontal m.
5. Oral orbicular m.
6. Parotidoauricular muscle
7. Masseter m.
8. Buccinator m.
9. Sternohyoid m.
10. Sternocephalic m.
11. Cleidocervical m.
12. Trapezius m.
13. Omotransverse m.
14. Clavicular tendon in brachiocephalic m.

15. Cleidobrachial m.
16. Deltoid m. (2 parts)
17. Brachialis m.
18. Brachial triceps m.
19. Deep pectoral m.
20. Widest m. of back (M. latissimus dorsi)
21. External abdominal oblique m.
22. Internal abdominal oblique m.
23. Sacrocaudal mm.
24. Superficial and middle gluteal mm.
25. Sartorial m.
26. Tensor m. of fascia lata
27. Femoral biceps m.
28. Semitendinous m.

Skeletal muscle is voluntary, i. e., under control of the will. Under a microscope, its fibers (cells) are striated (striped across) due to the arrangement of molecules within the fibers. The fibers of cardiac (heart) muscle are also striated, but the beating is involuntary. The third muscle type, smooth muscle, is nonstriated and its contractions are involuntary. Smooth muscle occurs in blood vessels, intestines, bladder, uterus, and erector muscles of hairs. Skeletal muscle accounts for 44% of body weight in most dogs, 57% in Greyhounds. Muscles function in locomotion, breathing, circulation, digestion, and reproduction. Muscles are also responsible for facial expression, hair raising, tail wagging, and barking.

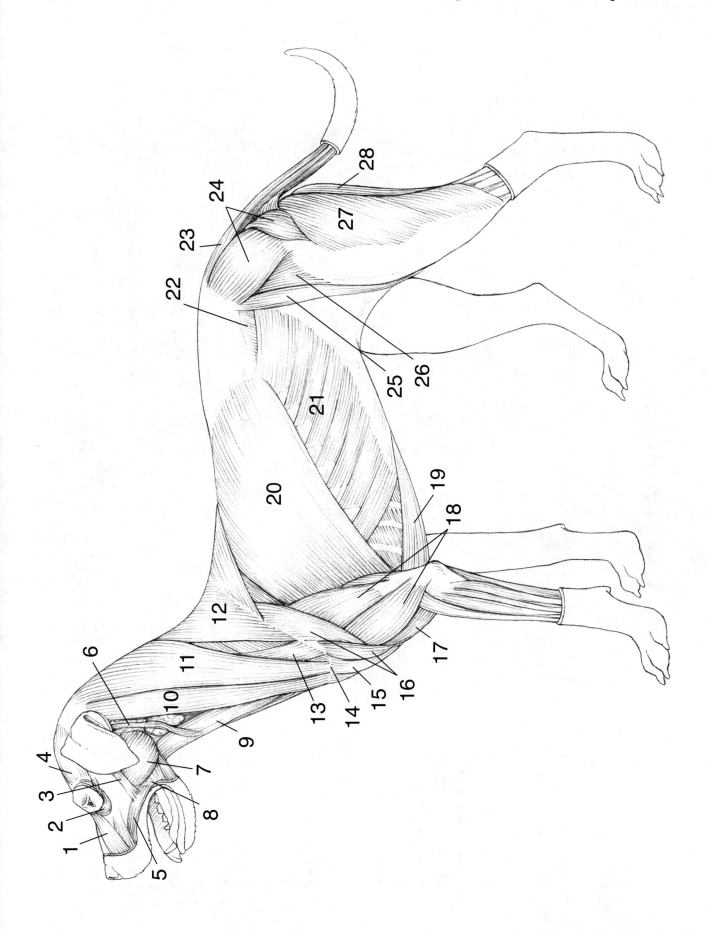

Deeper Muscles

PLATE 18

Figure 1. Left lateral view of deeper muscles of trunk and proximal parts of the limbs.   m. = muscle; mm. = muscles
Figure 2. Ventral view of muscles of shoulders and chest.

Underline the names below and color the muscles indicated on the drawings.

1. Splenius m.
2. Ventral serrated m.
3. Omotransverse m.
4. Sternocephalic m.
5. Rhomboid m.
6. Supraspinate m.
7. Infraspinate m.
8. Major teres m.
9. Deltoid m.
10. Brachial triceps m. (actually has 4 heads)
11. Brachial m.
12. Carpal and digital extensor mm.
13. Carpal and digital flexor mm.
14. Cranial dorsal serrated m.
15. Dorsal spinal and semispinal m.
16. Longest thoracic and lumbar m.
17. Iliocostal m.

18. External intercostal mm.
19. Transverse abdominal m.
20. Straight abdominal m.
21. Sartorial m.
22. Gluteal mm.
23. Femoral quadriceps m.
24. Adductor m.
25. Semimembranous m.
26. Semitendinous m.
27. Tarsal and digital extensor mm.
28. Tarsal and digital flexor mm.
29. Brachiocephalic m.
30. Sternocephalic m.
31. Sternohyoid mm.
32. Superficial pectoral m.
33. Deep pectoral m.
34. External abdominal oblique m.

Extensor muscles draw two members of a joint away from each other. The action is called extension.
Flexor muscles draw two members of a joint together. The action is called flexion.

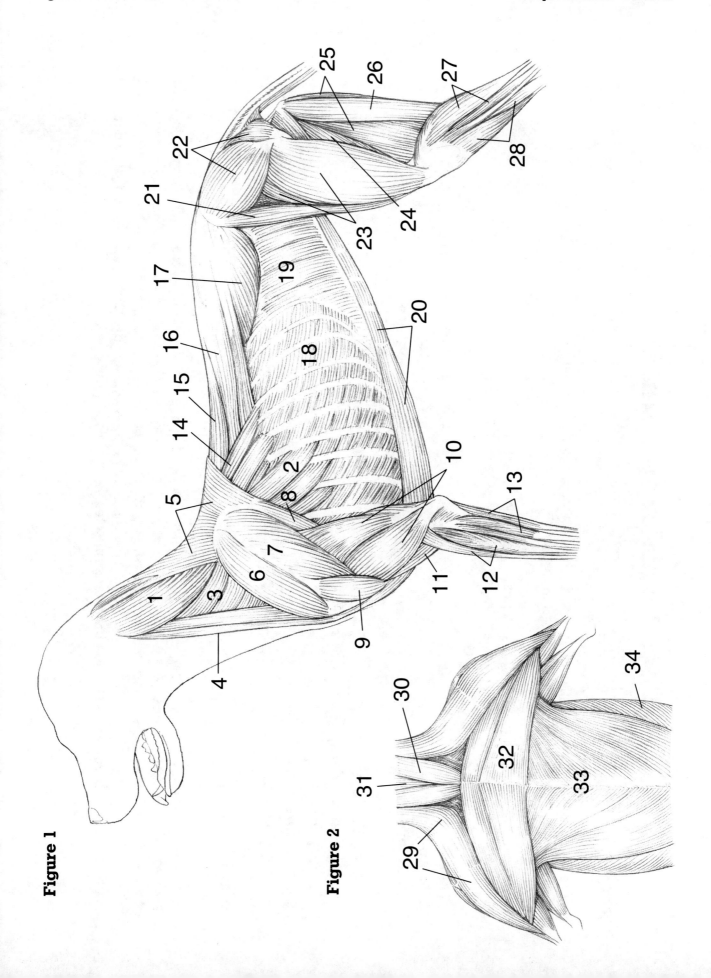

Figure 1

Figure 2

Deep Shoulder and Arm Muscles

PLATE 19

Figure 1. Lateral view of left shoulder and arm muscles. m. = muscle
Figure 2. Medial view of left shoulder and arm muscles. The limb is cut away from the trunk.

As you color the muscles indicated, try to determine their actions from their positions and the joints they cross. See the actions (results of muscular contractions) summarized in the paragraph below.

1. **Rhomboid m.**
2. **Ventral serrated m.**
   a. **Cranial part**
   b. **Caudal part**
3. **Widest dorsal m.**
   (M. latissimus dorsi)
4. **Deep pectoral m.**
5. **Supraspinate m.**
6. **Infraspinate m.**
7. **Major teres m.**
8. **Minor teres m.**

9. **Brachial triceps m.** (Lateral head removed)
   a. **Long head**
   b. **Accessory head**
   c. **Medial head**
10. **Brachial m.**
11. **Brachial biceps m.**
12. **Anconeal m.**
13. **Subscapular m.**
14. **Coracobrachial m.**
15. **Tensor m. of antebrachial fascia**

The **ventral serrated m.** supports the trunk. The forelimb is elevated by the **rhomboid m. Pectoral, supraspinate, coracobrachial** and **subscapular muscles** extend the shoulder joint; the **teres muscles** flex it and rotate the shoulder inward. The **infraspinate m.** rotates the shoulder outward and, with the **supraspinate m.,** serves as the lateral collateral ligament of the shoulder joint. The main extensor of the elbow, the **brachial triceps m.,** is aided by the **tensor m. of the fascia lata** and the **anconeal m.** The **brachial biceps** and **brachialis muscles** flex the elbow joint.

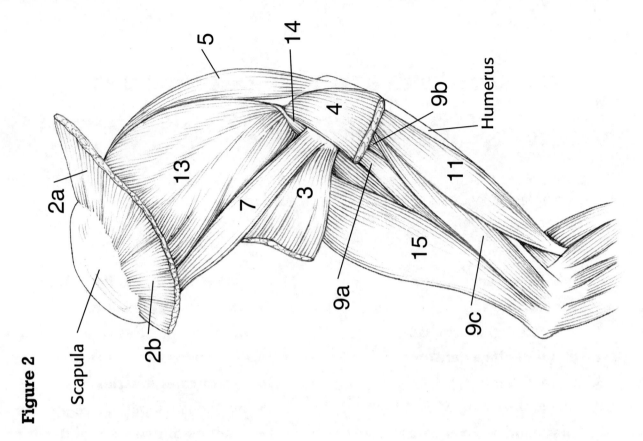

Figure 2

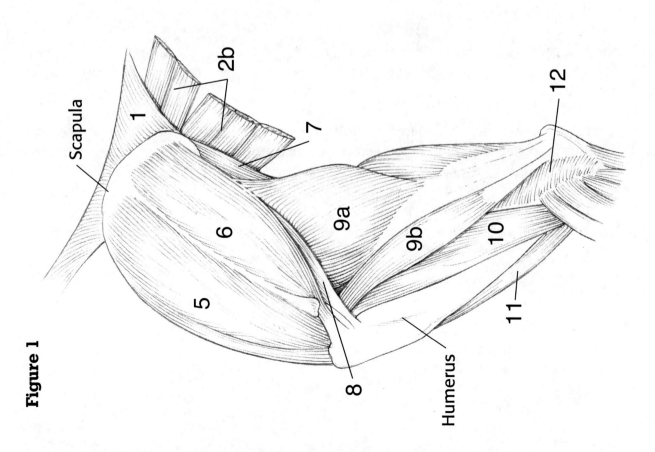

Figure 1

Forearm and Forefoot Muscles

PLATE 20

Dissections of left forearm and forefoot (forepaw) muscles and tendons attaching to the carpal bones, metacarpal bones and phalanges. m. = muscle

Underline the names below and color the muscles indicated on the plate.

1. **Radial carpal extensor m.**
2. **Pronator teres m.**
3. **Common digital extensor m.**
4. **Lateral digital extensor m.**
5. **Lateral ulnar m.**
6. **Long abductor m. of first digit**
7. **Ulnar head of ulnar carpal flexor m.**
8. **Humeral head of ulnar carpal flexor m.**
9. **Tendon of ulnar head of deep digital flexor m.**

10. **Superficial digital flexor m.**
11. **Radial carpal flexor m.**
12. **Abductor muscles of digits 1 and 5**
13. **4th interosseous muscle**
14. **Lumbricales muscles**
15. **Tendons of superficial digital flexor m.**
16. **Tendons of deep digital flexor m.**

An abductor muscle pulls a limb part away from the limb axis or a limb away from the trunk. The action is called abduction. The opposite term is adduction, the movement of a limb toward the trunk.

Pronator muscles rotate the forearm so that the palmar surface of the forepaw is directed laterad and thus to the ground (pronation). A **supinator muscle** (not seen here) acts to rotate the forearm so that the palmar surface of the paw is directed medially. This action, supination, is limited in the dog.

Notice that the tendons of the deep digital flexor m. perforate the tendons of the superficial digital flexor m. as they extend to their attachments on the digits.

Cranial view

Caudal view

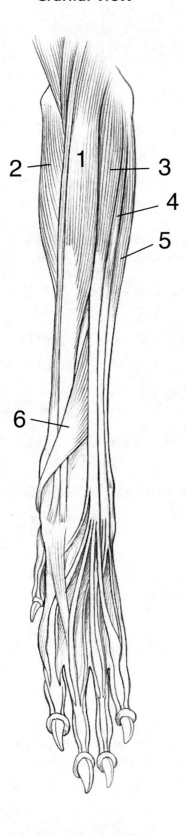

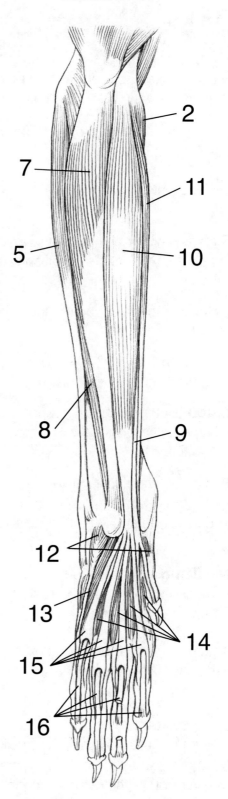

Forelimb Nerves

PLATE 21

Nerves supplying the forelimb muscles and sensation to the forelimb originate from the **brachial plexus**, a network formed by the ventral branches of the last three cervical and first two thoracic spinal nerves coming from the cervical swelling of the spinal cord.

The plate is a medial view of the left forelimb skeleton with the courses of the main forelimb nerves drawn roughly upon it.

Underline the names and trace the course of each nerve indicated by its matching number in a different color. n. = nerve

1. **Suprascapular n.** - around scapula to supply supraspinate and infraspinate muscles

2. **Subscapular n.** - supplies subscapular muscle

3. **Axillary n.** - to deltoid, major teres, minorteres and subscapular muscles

4. **Musculocutaneous n.** - supplies brachial biceps, coracobrachial and brachial muscles

5. **Radial n.** - to brachial triceps, radial carpal extensor, lateral ulnar, supinator and common and lateral digital extensor muscles

6. **Median n.** - supplies radial carpal flexor, superficial digital flexor, deep digital flexor and pronator muscles

7. **Caudal cutaneous antebrachial n.** - sensory to caudal forearm skin

8. **Medial cutaneous antebrachial n.** – sensory to medial forearm skin

9. **Cranial cutaneous antebrachial n.** - sensory to cranial forearm skin

10. **Ulnar n.** - supplies ulnar carpal flexor and deep digital flexor muscles

11. **Lateral cutaneous antebrachial n.** – sensory to lateral forearm skin

12. **Median sensory branches** - to caudal forearm and and palmar paw

13. **Ulnar sensory branches** - to palmar paw

14. **Superficial radial n.** – sensory to dorsal forearm and paw.

Other nerves from the brachial plexus supply the pectoral, brachiocephalic, ventral serrated, cutaneous trunk, and widest dorsal (latissimus dorsi) muscles, as well as the diaphragm via the phrenic nerve.

Injury to the **radial nerve** causes paralysis of the muscles it supplies. If it is damaged at the proximal end of the humerus, the forelimb cannot give support to the body because the brachial triceps cannot extend the elbow. Damage to the radial nerve in the region of the elbow results in lack of extension of the carpus and digits, and the dog supports its weight on the dorsal surface of the forefoot.

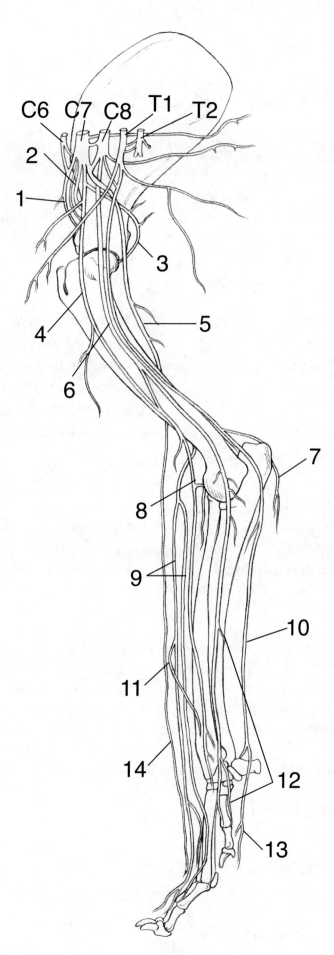

C6 C7 C8 T1 T2

2

1

3

4

5

6

7

8

9

10

11

14

12

13

Forelimb Blood Vessels

PLATE 22

In these drawings, the courses of the vessels are related roughly to the skeleton of the right forelimb. Dashed lines indicate the course of a vessel on the opposite side of the limb. Diameters of some of the smaller vessels are larger than normal to permit coloring. Underline the **boldfaced names** below and color names on the plate. Color the vessels indicated.

Major Arteries
1. **Thoracodorsal a.**
2. **Caudal circumflex humeral a.**
3. **Cranial circumflex humeral a.**
4. **Deep brachial a.**
5. **Bicipital a.**
6. **Superficial brachial a.**
7. **Cranial superficial antebrachial a. branches**
8. **Deep antebrachial a.**

Major Veins
9. **Thoracodorsal v.**
10. **Caudal circumflex humeral v.**
11. **Cran. circumflex humeral v.**
12. **Deep brachial v.**
13. **Bicipital v.**
14. **Deep antebrachial v.**

Blood reaches the forefoot primarily through the **axillary, brachial** and **median aa.** Secondary blood supplies are provided by the **common interosseous, caudal interosseous** and **radial aa.** and the **cranial superficial antebrachial a.** Arteries to the metacarpus and digits arise from the **superficial** and **deep palmar arches, cranial superficial antebrachial a.** and **dorsal carpal rete** (Latin, network).

Notice that most veins are satellites (Latin, *satelles* = companion) of arteries, but there are some differences between the venous drainage of the forelimb and its arterial supply. In addition to satellite veins, blood is drained from the forelimb by the **accessory cephalic, cephalic, median cubital** and **omobrachial vv.** The **cephalic** and **omobrachial vv.** carry blood to the external jugular v. The **cranial superficial antebrachial a.** and its **medial branch** lie on either side of the cephalic vein. Veins from the metacarpus and digits return blood to the **proximal** and **distal palmar venous arches** and the **accessory cephalic v.**

Veins differ from arteries in that they:
    a. contain a larger volume of blood.
    b. have thinner walls.
    c. usually have valves. The cusps of valves direct blood toward the heart.

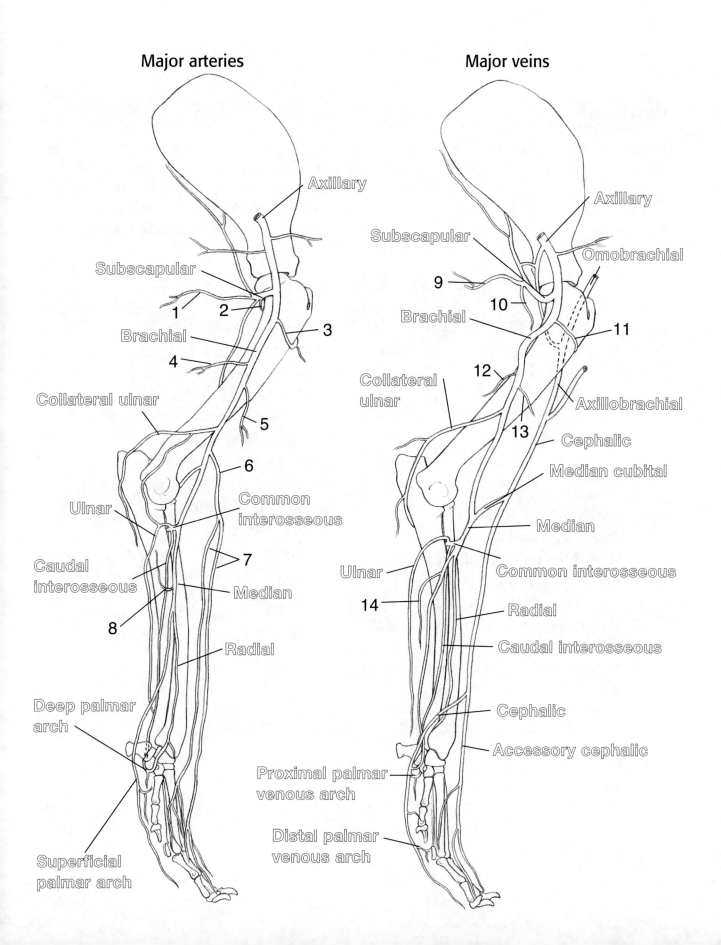

Major arteries

Axillary

Subscapular

1
2
3

Brachial
4

Collateral ulnar

5

6

Ulnar

Common
interosseous

Caudal
interosseous

7

8

Median

Radial

Deep palmar
arch

Superficial
palmar arch

Major veins

Axillary

Subscapular

Omobrachial

9

10

Brachial

11

Collateral
ulnar

12

13

Axillobrachial

Cephalic

Median cubital

Median

Common interosseous

Ulnar

Radial

14

Caudal interosseous

Cephalic

Accessory cephalic

Proximal palmar
venous arch

Distal palmar
venous arch

The Dog's Feet (Paws)

PLATE 23

The terms, foot and paw, have been used interchangeably. On Plate 1, notice that the forefoot or forepaw (L., *manus*, hand) consists of the carpus, metacarpus, and digits; the hindfoot or hindpaw (L. *pes*, foot) consists of the tarsus, metatarsus, and digits. Most dog experts consider only the distal parts of the metacarpus or metatarsus and the digits to be the paw. The pastern includes the metacarpus or metatarsus. On Plate 7, notice the position of the articulated bones of the feet. On Plate 13, the bones are slightly disarticulated.

Underline the **boldfaced names** below and color the structures indicated

Figure 1.
a. Palmar view of left forefoot. The **carpal pad** (stopper pad) touches the ground only when a rapidly running dog corners.
b. Palmar view of the left hindfoot. There is no pad over the tarsus.

Figure 2.
a. Superficial palmar dissection of left forefoot with footpads intact.
 1. **Superficial muscles of paw.**
 2. **Branching tendons of superficial digital flexor muscle**
b. Deeper palmar dissection of left forefoot.
 3. **Branching tendons of deep digital flexor muscle**
 4. **Branching tendons of superficial digital flexor muscle (cut)**
 (Branching digital extensor tendons attach dorsally.)

Figure 3.
Axial section of a digit.
 1. **Horny wall of claw**
 2. **Dermis**
 3. **Ungual process of distal phalanx**
 4. **Dorsal elastic ligament**
 5. **Distal sesamoid bone**
 6. **Deep digital flexor m. tendon**
 7. **Middle phalanx**
 8. **Proximal phalanx**
 9. **Digital footpad** – highly cornified epidermis and fibrofatty tissue with merocrine sweat glands in subcutis. Papillae project from the surface of the footpad.

TRIMMING A DOG'S CLAWS: Claws grow from the epidermal matrix at the base at an average rate of l.9 mm per week. If they are not worn down naturally, they should be trimmed. Align the cutting edge of the claw trimmer with the surface of the digital pad. In nonpigmented claws the blood in the dermis can be seen.

Figure 1

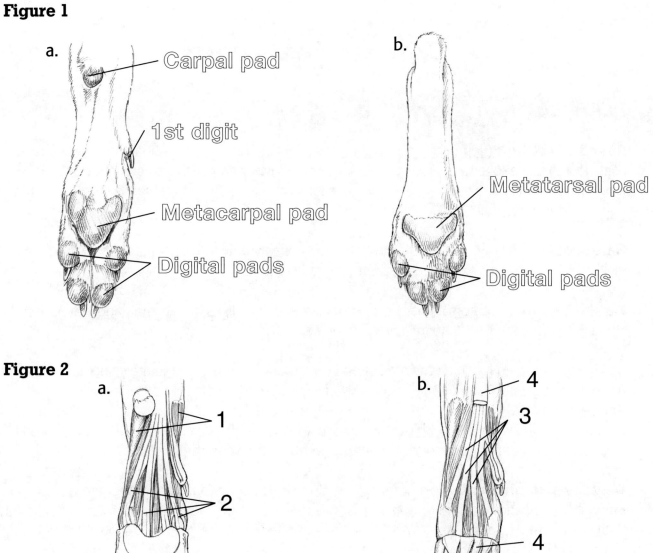

a.
Carpal pad
1st digit
Metacarpal pad
Digital pads

b.
Metatarsal pad
Digital pads

Figure 2

a.
1
2

b.
4
3
4

Figure 3

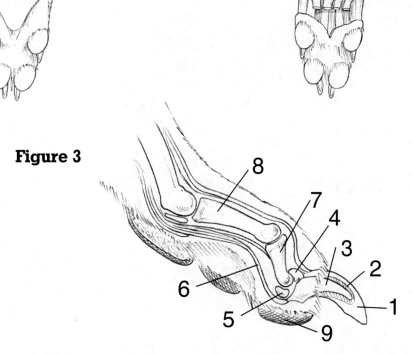

8
7
4
3
2
1
6
5
9

Types of Feet (Paws)

PLATE 24

Round or cat foot (<u>compact</u> <u>foot,</u> <u>close-cupped</u> <u>foot</u>). This foot is compact with well-arched digits (toes) close together. Digits 3 and 4 are only slightly longer than digits 2 and 5. The footprint is circular. An <u>oval</u> <u>foot</u> is similar except that digits 3 and 4 are somewhat longer than in a round foot, leaving an oval footprint.

Hare foot (<u>rabbit</u> <u>paw</u>). Digits 3 and 4 are considerably longer than digits 2 and 5, and the digits are less arched. The footprint is an elongated oval.

Flat foot (<u>down</u> <u>in</u> <u>pastern</u>). Instead of being arched, the digits are straight, and the pastern slopes appreciably. The footprint is very elongated.

Splay foot (<u>spread</u> <u>foot</u>). Digits are set apart from one another. Moderately spreading feet are normal for the Irish Water Spaniel, but they are considered a defect in other breeds.
Snowshoe foot. This is an oval foot with well-arched digits and well-cornified (horny) and thick footpads. Well-developed <u>webbing</u> and fur occur between the digits. Water-retrieving breeds as well as mountain and arctic dogs have strong webbing between the digits.

Dewclaws on hindfoot. Whereas single or double dewclaws on the hindfeet are uncommon in most breeds, they occur more often in some (Saint Bernard, Newfoundland, Chesapeake Bay Retriever). In most dogs, dewclaws should be removed from the hindfeet. However, they are not removed from the Briard and Great Pyrenees , since they are a show requirement in these breeds.

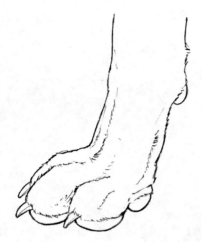

Round or cat foot

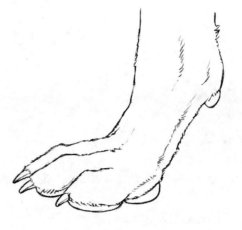

Hare foot

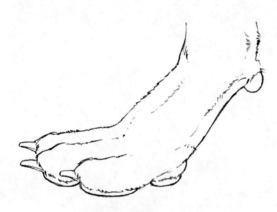

Flat foot
(down in pastern)

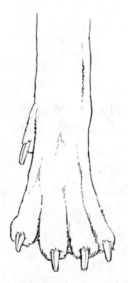

Splay foot

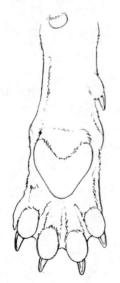

Snowshoe foot

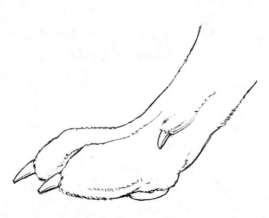

Dewclaw on hindfoot

Bones of the Pelvis

PLATE 25

Figure 1. Dorsocaudal view of bony pelvis.

Color in the names of the bones and the bones indicated.

Each **hip bone** (os coxae) consists of the fused **ilium, ischium** (pronounced iskium), **pubis** and **acetabular bone**. The two hip bones are joined at the **pelvic symphysis**. The **sacrum** articulates with each **ilium** at a sacroiliac **joint**.

Figure 2. Left lateral view of mature bony pelvis.

Underline the following names and color the parts of the bones indicated:
1. **Crest of ilium**
2. **Cranial dorsal iliac spine**
3. **Caudal dorsal iliac spine**
4. **Iliopubic eminence**
5. **Ischiatic spine**
6. **Obturator foramen**
7. **Ischiatic tuber**
8. **Pelvic symphysis**
9. **Pecten of pubis**
10. **Sacroiliac joints**
11. **Cranial ventral iliac spine**
12. **Caudal ventral iliac spine**
13. **Acetabulum -** consists of a semicircular articular surface, the <u>lunate face</u>, surrounding a deep <u>acetabular fossa</u>.

Figure 3. Developing **hip bone** of a puppy. Cartilage is stippled. The small **acetabular bone** fuses with the **ilium, ischium** and **pubis** to form the **acetabulum** (socket of the hip joint). Fusion is completed in the 12th week after birth.

Figure 1

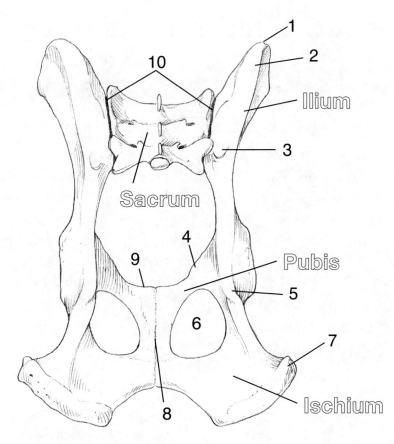

1
2
Ilium
10
3
Sacrum
4
9
Pubis
5
6
7
8
Ischium

Figure 2

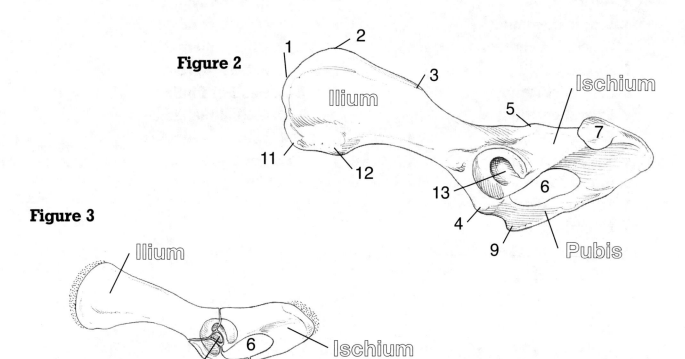

1
2
3
Ischium
Ilium
5
7
11
13
6
12
4
9
Pubis

Figure 3

Ilium
6
Ischium
Acetabular bone
Pubis

Bones of the Thigh and Leg

PLATE 26

Color in the names on the drawing and the bones indicated in different colors.

A. Cranial view of left **femur**. The **patella** is a large sesamoid bone attached to the femoral quadriceps muscle and its tendon. It slides proximad and distad (up and down) on the **trochlea**. Parapatellar cartilages (stippled) on each side increase the articular surface area.

B. Caudal view of left **femur**. The ligament of the head of the femur attaches in the **fovea**. Two small **sesamoid bones** (fabellae) in the medial and lateral heads of the gastrocnemius muscle articulate with the **medial** and **lateral condyles** of the femur. A third even smaller **sesamoid bone** is in the tendon of origin of the popliteal muscle and articulates with the lateral condyle.

C. Cranial view of left **tibia** and **fibula**.

D. Caudal view of left **tibia** and **fibula**.

Underline names and color the following parts of the:

Femur

1. **Head**
2. **Neck**
3. **Lesser trochanter**
4. **Greater trochanter**
5. **Trochlea**
6. **Medial epicondyle**
7. **Lateral epicondyle**
8. **Fovea**
9. **Trochanteric fossa**
10. **Intertrochanteric crest**
11. **Supracondylar tuberosities**
12. **Lateral condyle**
13. **Medial condyle**

Tibia and **Fibula**

14. **Medial condyle**
15. **Intercondylar eminence**
16. **Lateral condyle**
17. **Tibial tuberosity**
18. **Extensor groove**
19. **Head of fibula**
20. **Medial malleolus**
21. **Lateral malleolus**
22. **Cochlea** – lateral - oblique grooves

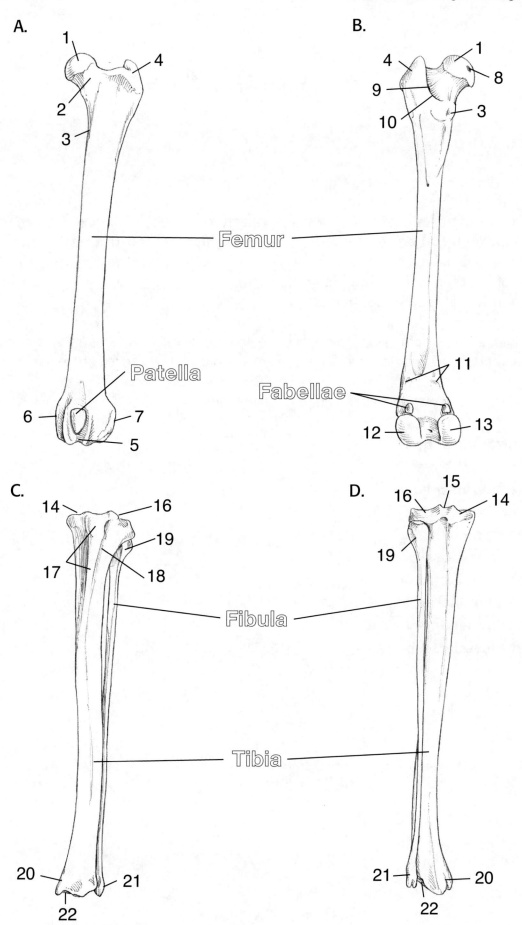

A.

1
4
2
3

Femur

Patella

6
7
5

B.

4
1
9
8
10
3

Femur

11
Fabellae
12
13

C.

14
16
19
17
18

Fibula

Tibia

20
21
22

D.

16
15
14
19

Fibula

Tibia

21
20
22

Bones of the Tarsus

PLATE 27

Lateral, dorsal, and plantar views of the bones of the left tarsus.

There are seven bones in the tarsus (hock): **calcaneus** (fibular tarsal bone), **talus** (tibial tarsal bone), **central tarsal bone** and the **first, second, third** and **fourth tarsal bones**. More than three times as long as the carpus, the hock includes the talocrural (ankle) joint between the cochlea of the **tibia** and the **trochlea** of the **talus** and tarsometatarsal joints between **tarsal bones I** to **IV** and **metatarsal bones 1** to **5**.

Except for the shape of the first metatarsal bone and the usual absence of a first digit, the metatarsal bones and phalanges are similar to the metacarpal bones and phalanges of the forefoot.

Underline the following names and color the bones and their parts:

CT. Central tarsal bone
  I. First tarsal bone
  II. Second tarsal bone
III. Third tarsal bone
 IV. Fourth tarsal bone
  1. First metatarsal bone
  2. Second metatarsal bone
  3. Third metatarsal bone
  4. Fourth metatarsal bone
  5. Fifth metatarsal bone

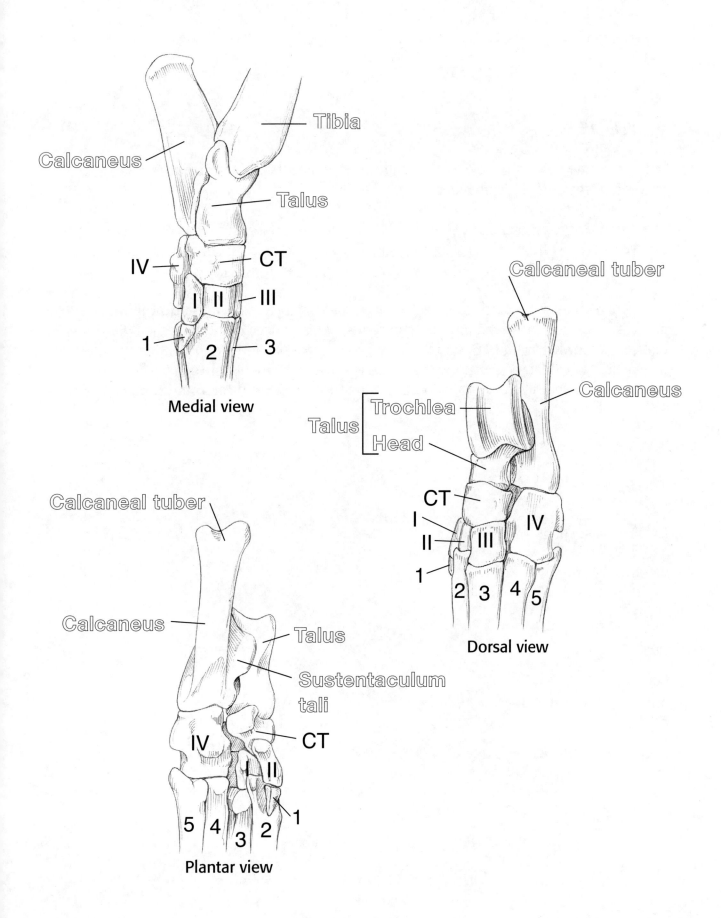

Calcaneus

Tibia

Talus

IV

CT

I II III

1

2 3

Medial view

Calcaneal tuber

Talus {
Trochlea

Head

Calcaneus

CT

I

II III

IV

1

2 3 4 5

Dorsal view

Calcaneal tuber

Calcaneus

Talus

Sustentaculum tali

IV

CT

I II

1

5 4 3 2

Plantar view

Joints of the Hindlimb

PLATE 28

Color in the names of the joints and the arrows indicating the **flexor surfaces** of the joints. The angles become smaller when the joints are flexed.

The **sacroiliac joint** on each side is formed by articular surfaces on the wing of the ilium and the wing of the sacrum. It is a stabilizing joint in which the articular surfaces are covered with fibrocartilage and supported by dorsal and ventral sacroiliac ligaments.

Among the joints of the hock, the greatest movement occurs in the **talocrural joint**. The grooves in the cochlea of the tibia and the corresponding ridges of the trochlea of the talus are directed somewhat laterad. Due to this arrangement, the hindfeet are pushed past the outside of the forefeet when the dog is galloping. There is some movement between the talus and calcaneus, but very little movement occurs in the **intertarsal** and **tarsometatarsal joints**.

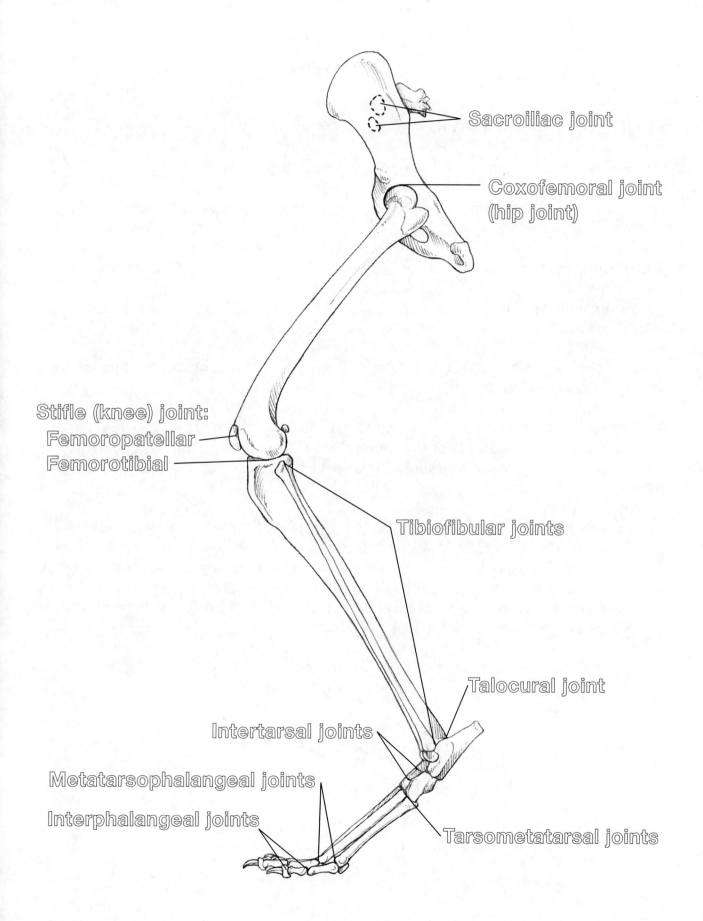

Sacroiliac joint

Coxofemoral joint
(hip joint)

Stifle (knee) joint:
Femoropatellar
Femorotibial

Tibiofibular joints

Talocural joint

Intertarsal joints

Metatarsophalangeal joints

Interphalangeal joints

Tarsometatarsal joints

Hip Joint

PLATE 29

Ventral view of a dog's bony pelvis and hip joints, including major ligaments.

Underline the numbered names below and fill in the names on the plates. Color the structures indicated in the same colors.

1. Seventh lumbar vertebra
2. Sacrum
3. First caudal vertebra
4. Ischiatic tuber

Most ligaments function in holding bones together in joints. The **sacrotuberous ligament** is a structure of origin for major muscles over the hip.

The left **hip joint** (coxofemoral joint) is normal. The extent of the **articular capsule** is indicated by a dashed line. The **ligament of the femoral head** binds the head of the femur to the acetabulum. The **transverse acetabular ligament** bridges the notch in the acetabulum, completing the fibrocartilaginous acetabular lip.

A **dysplastic hip joint** is seen on the right. Hip dysplasia (from the Greek, dys-, abnormal + plassein, to form) is an inherited developmental condition in which the head of the femur and the acetabulum do not articulate properly. It may occur in fast growing puppies of large breeds such as the German Shepherd Dog, Labrador Retriever and Rottweiler. The condition is noticed as a painful hip in later life. Diagnosis may be made through manipulation of the hip joint by a veterinarian and confirmed by radiographs (X-ray films).

An early corrective measure involves a triple pinning of each ilium. Total hip replacement may be the only surgical option in mature dogs afflicted with hip dysplasia.

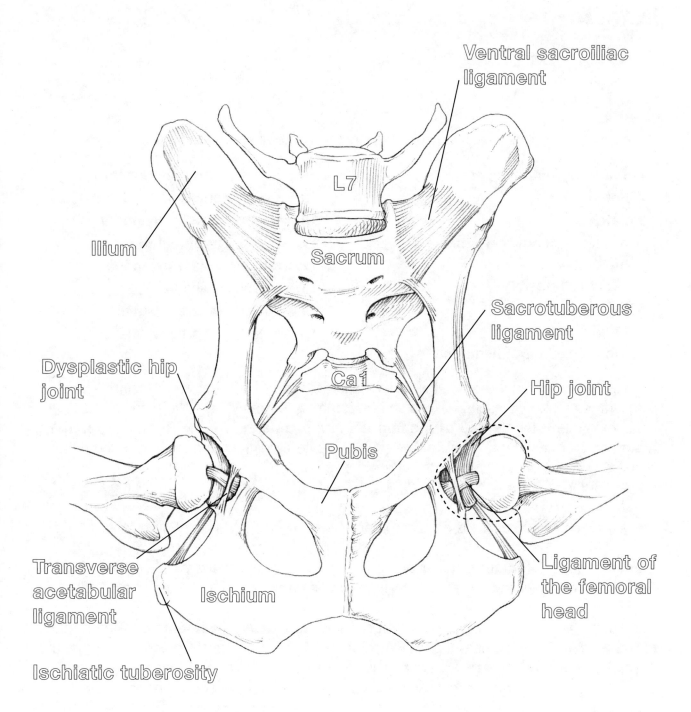

Ventral sacroiliac ligament

Ilium

L7

Sacrum

Sacrotuberous ligament

Dysplastic hip joint

Ca1

Hip joint

Pubis

Transverse acetabular ligament

Ischium

Ligament of the femoral head

Ischiatic tuberosity

Stifle Joint

PLATE 30

Dissections of a dog's left stifle (knee) joint.
A. Medial view   **B.** Lateral view
C. Cranial view   **D.** Caudal view

Underline the following terms and color the structures indicated on the drawing.

1. Tendon - fem. quadriceps m.
2. Patella
3. Patellar ligament
   (continues **tendon of fem. quadriceps m.** to **4.**)
4. Tibial tuberosity
5. Fabellae
6. Medial meniscus
7. Medial collateral ligament

8. Tendon - long dig. ext. m.
9. Lateral meniscus
10. Lateral collateral ligament
11. Tendon - popliteal muscle
12. Cranial cruciate ligament
13. Transverse ligament
14. Caudal cruciate ligament
15. Meniscofemoral ligament

There are two joints in the stifle - the femoropatellar joint and the femorotibial joint. A single, compartmented joint capsule (dashed line) is common to both joints. The **patella** is a large sesamoid bone in the **tendon of the femoral quadriceps m.** with the continuing **patellar ligament** attaching to the **tibial tuberosity**. The patella riding on the trochlea of the femur changes direction of pull by the femoral quadriceps muscle, resulting in extension of the femorotibial joint.

Patellar luxation (dislocation) is most common in toy breeds such as the Pomeranian.

Medial and **lateral menisci** (plural of meniscus) are C-shaped plates of fibrocartilage between the femoral condyles and the tibial condyles, providing more congruent articular surfaces.

Named for their tibial attachments, **cranial** and **caudal cruciate ligaments** cross each other as they extend from the femur to the tibia. A common cause of hindlimb lameness is rupture of the **cranial cruciate ligament**, increasing cranial movement of the tibia. Several surgical procedures including extra-articular (outside the joint) fixation and intra-articular (inside the joint) replacement of the ligament are employed to correct the lameness. In a procedure called tibial plateau leveling osteotomy (TPLO), the proximal end of the tibia is rotated. As a result of this procedure, when the tibial condyles (the plateau) move against the femoral condyles, the joint is stabilized.

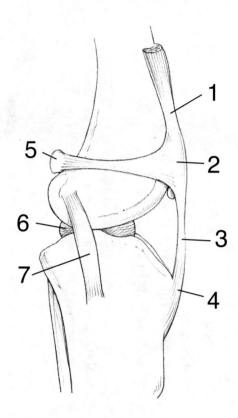

A. Medial view

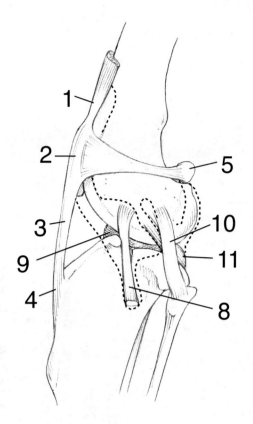

B. Lateral view

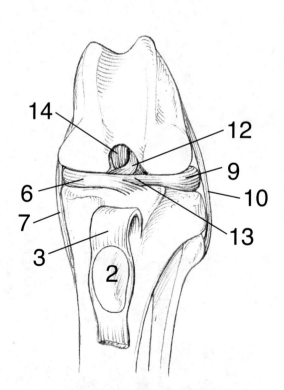

C. Cranial view

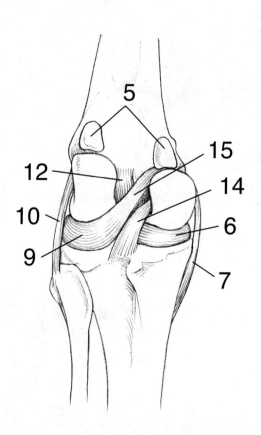

D. Caudal view

Dog Anatomy - A Coloring Atlas

Hindlimb Muscles - Lateral Views

PLATE 31

Figure 1. Lateral view of superficial muscles of left hip and thigh.
Figure 2. Lateral view of deep dissection of left hindlimb muscles.

As you color the muscles, try to determine their actions from their positions and the joints they cross. See below.

1. Femoral biceps m.
2. Semitendinous m.
3. Semimembranous m.
4. Superficial gluteal m.
5. Middle gluteal m.
6. Tensor of fascia lata m.
7. Sartorial m.
8. Deep gluteal m.
9. Femoral quadriceps m.
   a. Femoral straight m.
   b. Lateral vast m.
10. Sacrotuberous ligament
11. Tendon of int. obturator on gemelli muscles
12. Femoral quadrate m.
13. Adductor m.

14. Caudal crural abductor m.
15. Gastrocnemius m.
16. Deep digital flexor m.
17. Cranial tibial m.
18. Long peroneal m.
19. Long digital extensor m.
20. Common calcanean tendon
21. Tendon of long digital ext.
22. Tendon of lat. digital ext.
23. Tendon of long peroneal m.
24. Tendon of short peroneal m.
25. Tendon of superficial digital flexor m.
26. Fifth interosseous m.
27. Termination of tendon of deep digital flexor m.
28. Lateral short digital extensor m.

The gluteal group of muscles (**superficial, middle** and **deep gluteal muscles** and the **tensor of the fascia lata**) extend the hip and help abduct the hip joint. Insertions of the hamstring group (**femoral biceps, semitendinous** and **semimembranous muscles**) attach proximal and distal to the stifle joint. Tendons from the femoral biceps and semitendinous muscles join tendons of the **superficial digital flexor** and **gastrocnemius** to form the **common calcanean tendon**. The main action of the hamstring group is extension of the hip joint. Depending on the location of the muscles and the position of the foot on or or off the ground, other actions are flexion or extension of the stifle and extension of the hock. The **internal obturator** and **gemelli muscles** rotate the hip outward. The **long peroneal muscle** flexes the hock and turns the foot outward. The **cranial tibial muscle** also flexes the hock but turns the foot inward.

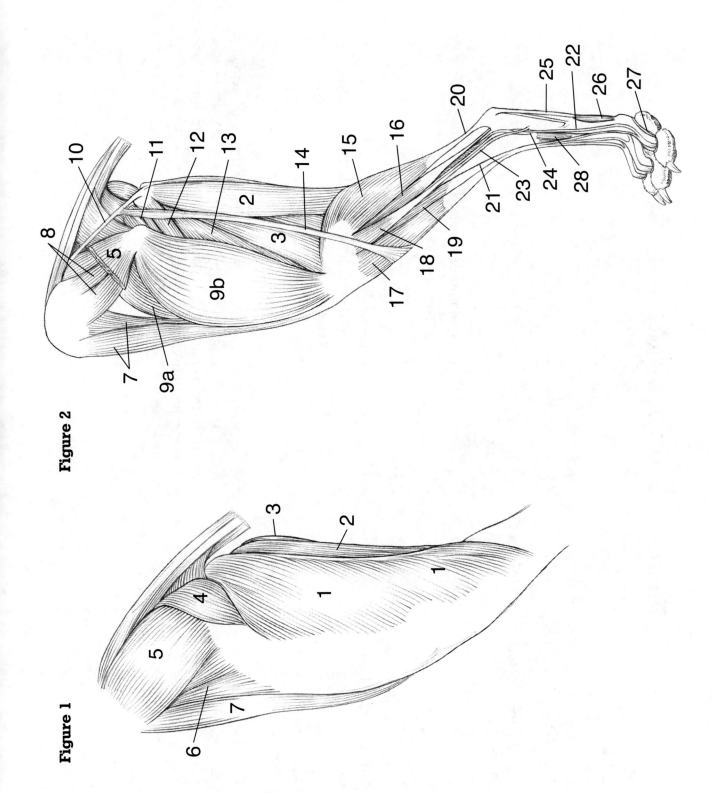

Figure 2

Figure 1

Hindlimb Muscles - Medial Views

PLATE 32

Figure 1. Medial view of superficial muscles of left hindlimb.
Figure 2. Medial view of deep muscles of left hindlimb. m. = muscle.

As you color the muscles indicated, try to visualize their actions from their positions and the joints that they cross. See paragraph below.

1. **Sartorial m.**
   a. Cranial part
   b. Caudal part
2. **Femoral quadriceps m.**
   a. Femoral straight m.
   b. Medial vast m.
3. **Pectineal m.**
4. **Adductor m.**
5. **Gracilis m.**

6. **Semimembranous m.**
7. **Semitendinous m.**
8. **Gastrocnemius m.**
9. **Superficial digital flexor m.**
10. **Deep digital flexor m.**
11. **Calcanean tendon (Achilles tendon)**
12. **Cranial tibial m.**
13. **Popliteal m.**

Inserting on the tibial tuberosity by means of the patellar ligament, the four-headed **femoral quadriceps muscle** is the principal extensor of the stifle. The cranial part of the **sartorial muscle** and the cranial part of the **semimembranous muscle** also extend the stifle. Flexors of the stifle include the caudal part of the **sartorial muscle,** the caudal part of the **semimembranous muscle,** and the **semitendinous, gracilis popliteal** and **gastrocnemius muscles.** Adduction of the hindlimb is done by the **pectineal,** adductor and gracilis muscles. The deep digital flexor muscle consists of the **long digital flexor** and the long **flexor of the hallux** (L., hallux = great toe, the 1st digit of the hindfoot, the rarely present dewclaw).

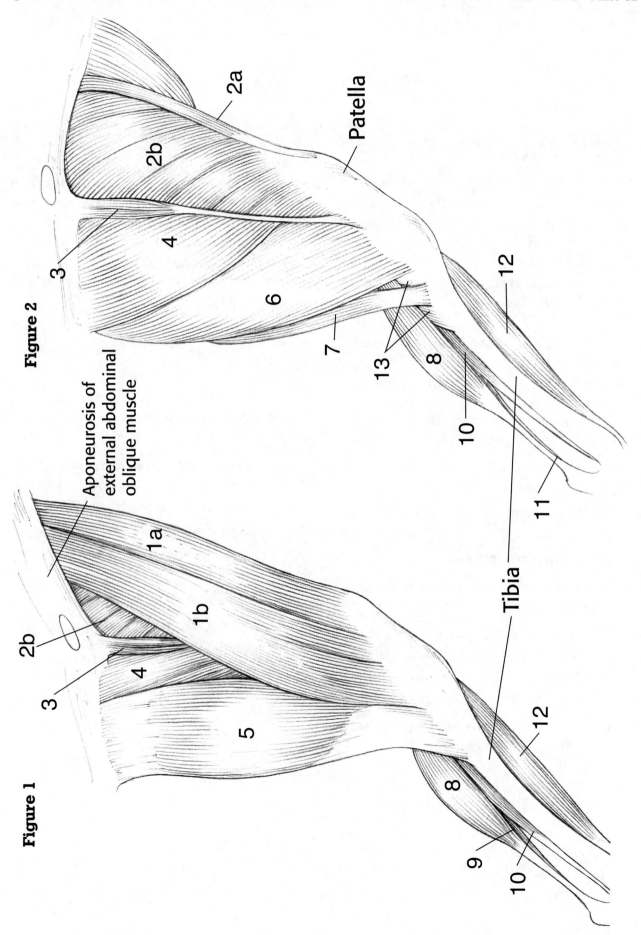

Figure 2

2a

2b

Patella

3

4

6

7

13

8

10

11

12

Aponeurosis of
external abdominal
oblique muscle

Figure 1

2b

3

4

1a

1b

5

Tibia

8

9

10

12

Hindlimb Nerves

PLATE 33

Hindlimb nerves arise from the **lumbosacral plexus**, a network on each side formed by the ventral branches of the last four lumbar nerves and the three sacral nerves. Interconnections among these nerves are variable. In addition to contributing to hindlimb nerves, sacral nerves also give origin to nerves supplying pelvic organs. The **femoral** and **obturator nerves** arise from **lumbar nerves 4** through **6**. **Lumbar nerves 6** and **7** and **sacral nerves 1** and **2** form the **lumbosacral trunk**, which gives off a branch to the small hip muscles and the **cranial** and **caudal gluteal nerves** and then continues as the **sciatic nerve.**

Medial view of left hindlimb skeleton with courses of nerves related roughly to regions of the hindlimb. Underline the names below and trace the course of each nerve in a different color. n. = nerve; m. = muscle.

1. **Femoral n.** - supplies sublumbar muscles and femoral quadriceps m.

2. **Saphenous n.** - to sartorial m.; sensory to medial side of hindlimb.

3. **Obturator n.** - supplies adductor muscles of hip.

4. **Lumbosacral trunk**

5. **Cranial and caudal gluteal nn.** - to flexor and extensor muscles of hip.

6. **Caudal cutaneus femoral n.** - sensory to skin of caudal thigh.

7. **Sciatic n.** - motor to hamstring muscles; sensory to hindlimb via its branches.

8. **Lateral cutaneous sural n.** - sensory to skin of lateral leg region.

9. **Common peroneal n.** - motor branch to femoral biceps m.

10. **Superficial peroneal n.** - supplies lateral digital extensor m.; sensory to skin over dorsal aspect of leg and foot.

11. **Deep peroneal n.** - to dorsolateral muscles of leg; sensory to foot.

12. **Tibial n.** - to hamstring, gastrocnemius, popliteal and caudal crural mm.

13. **Caudal cutaneous sural n.** - sensory to caudal skin of leg and hock.

14. **Medial plantar n.** - to medial aspect of foot.

15. **Lateral plantar n.** - to lateral and middle aspects of foot.

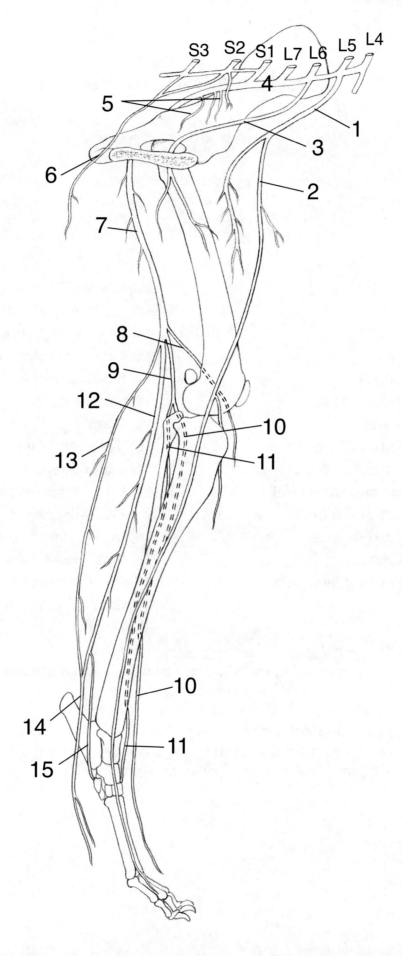

Hindlimb Blood Vessels

PLATE 34

Medial views of the vessels related roughly to the skeleton of the left hindlimb. Color the names and the courses of the vessels, using red for arteries and blue for veins. The diameter of some of the vessels is larger than normal to permit coloring.

a. = artery, v. = vein

Major Arteries

1. Aorta
2. Internal iliac a.
3. Iliolumbar a.
4. Cranial gluteal a.
5. Internal pudendal a.
6. Deep femoral a.
7. Pudendoepigastric trunk
8. Medial circumflex femoral a.
9. Lateral circumflex femoral a.
10. Descending genicular a.
11. Distal caudal femoral a.
12. Caudal tibial a.
13. Cr. branch of saphenous a.

Major Veins

14. Ca. branch of saphenous a.
15. Perforating metatarsal a.
16. Caudal caval vein
17. Internal iliac v.
18. Iliolumbar v.
19. Cranial gluteal v.
20. Deep femoral v.
21. Pudendoepigastric trunk
22. Lat. circumflex femoral v.
23. Medial saphenous v.
24. Descending genicular v.
25. Distal caudal femoral v.
26. Cranial branches of saphenous veins
27. Caudal branches of saphenous veins

Blood flows to the metatarsal and digital arteries of the hindfoot primarily through the following sequence of arteries: **external iliac - femoral - popliteal - cranial tibial - dorsal pedal** and **saphenous**.

Branches of the **saphenous a.** supply the skin: the caudal branch gives origin to the plantar common digital aa. The **perforatng metatarsal a.** and plantar arteries (from the **saphenous a.**) form a deep plantar arch that gives origin to plantar metatarsal aa.

Most veins are satellites (Latin, *satelles* = companion) of arteries.

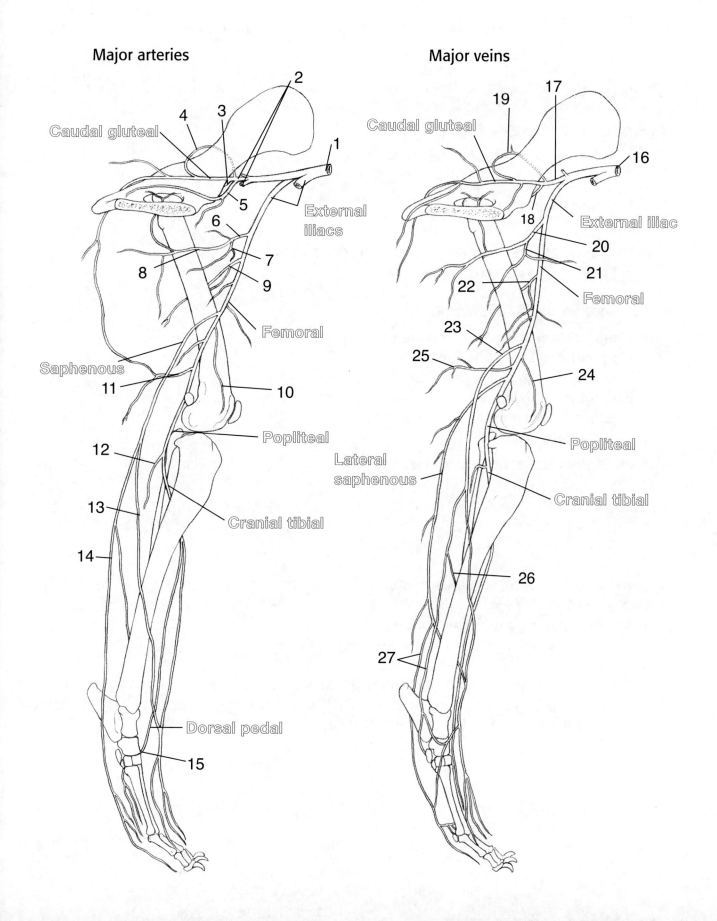

Major arteries

2
3
4
Caudal gluteal
1
5
External iliacs
6
7
8
9
Femoral
Saphenous
11
10
Popliteal
12
13
Cranial tibial
14
Dorsal pedal
15

Major veins

19
17
Caudal gluteal
16
18
External iliac
20
21
Femoral
22
23
25
24
Popliteal
Lateral saphenous
Cranial tibial
26
27

Back and Neck Muscles

PLATE 35

Figure 1. Epaxial muscle systems. Lateral views.

Using three different colors, fill in the diagrammatic drawings of the:

  I. Iliocostal muscle system – lateral group of muscles
   1. Lumbar iliocostal m.
   2. Thoracic iliocostal m.

 II. Longest (Longissimus) muscle system – intermediate group of muscles
   3. Longest thoracic and lumbar m.
   4. Longest cervical m.
   5. Longest capital (head) m.

III. Transversospinal muscle system – medial group of muscles
   6. Spinal and semispinal muscles
   7. Splenius m. (cut and reflected)
   8. Capital semispinal m. – Formed by the two muscles below.
    a. Cervical biventer m.
    b. Complexus m.

   Multifidus and rotator muscles – not seen here; deeper, beween vertebrae

Epaxial muscles lie dorsal to the vertebral transverse processes. Working together, they extend the neck and back; on one side, they produce lateral movement. Hypaxial muscles are located ventral to the vertebral bodies and tranverse processes.

Figure 2. Sublumbar muscles (ventral to last three thoracic and the lumbar vertebrae).
Ventral view of muscles on the left side. Also considered with muscles of the pelvic limb.
  1. Lumbar quadrate m. – fixes lumbar vertebral column
  2. Minor psoas m. – flexes lumbar vertebral column
  3. Major psoas m.
  4. Iliacus m. – This muscle and the **major psoas m.** fuse to form the **iliopsoas m.,** the primary flexor of the hip. If the femur is fixed, it flexes the vertebral column. If the pelvic limb is extended caudad, the trunk is pulled caudad.

Figure 1

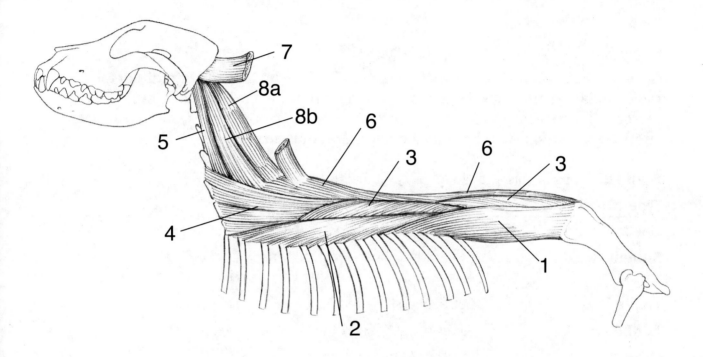

Figure 2

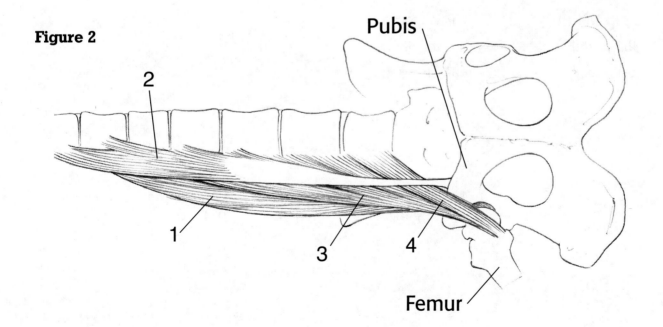

Tails

PLATE 36

Figure 1. Tail muscles.

Locate and color the tail muscles. m. = muscle.

The dog's tail is elevated (extended) by contraction of the **medial** and **lateral dorsal sacrocaudal muscles**; the tail is depressed (flexed) by the **medial** and **lateral ventral sacrocaudal muscles**; and it is flexed laterad (to the side or "wagged") by the **caudal intertransversarius**, **anal levator**, and **coccygeal muscles**.

Figure 2. Types of tails. Color the tails and their names.

Type of Tail	Examples
Gay tail	Many terriers. Tail docked (shortened by cutting)
Bobtail	Old English Sheepdog, Doberman Pinscher A very short tail, either natural or docked
Plumed tail	Collie, English Setter
Curled tail	Siberian Husky and other Northern breeds, Pug
Otter tail	Labrador Retriever
Ring at end tail	Afghan Hound
Screw tail	Bulldog, Boston Terrier
Snap tail	Pekingnese
Sickle tail	Otter Hound
Whip tail	Dachshund

Figure 1

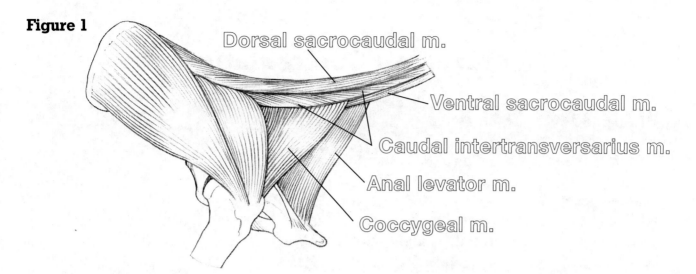

Dorsal sacrocaudal m.

Ventral sacrocaudal m.

Caudal intertransversarius m.

Anal levator m.

Coccygeal m.

Figure 2

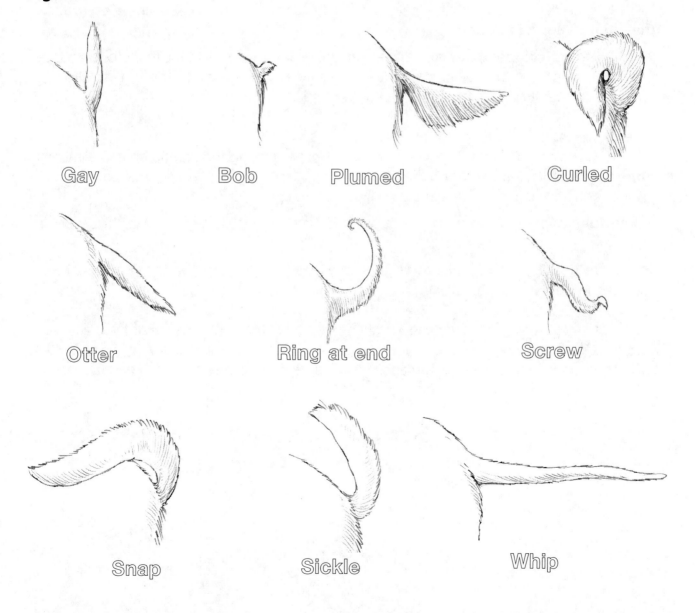

Gay

Bob

Plumed

Curled

Otter

Ring at end

Screw

Snap

Sickle

Whip

Forelimb Conformation

PLATE 37

Color the dashed lines from **p** (proximal) to **d** (distal).

Cranial views: A

A line dropped from the point of the shoulder (middle of the shoulder joint) to the ground bisects a forelimb with **normal (straight) conformation**.

In **base narrow (too narrow in front) conformation**, the feet are often directed laterad (outward), so-called **east-west feet**.

Laterally projecting elbows with the feet placed wide apart are seen in the **base wide (out at the elbows) conformation**.

In **fiddle front (chippendale) conformation**, the elbows project laterad, the forearm slopes mediad (inward), and the sloping pasterns and feet are directed laterad. This conformation causes excessive strain on the medial side of the carpus.

Lateral views: B

Laterally, a line dropped from the middle of the scapular spine to the ground on a forelimb with **normal (straight) conformation** bisects the limb as far as the carpus and then drops just plantar (behind) the foot to the ground.

In **knuckled over conformation**, the carpus buckles dorsad (foreward), causing the metacarpus to deviate palmarad (rearward).

The **down in the pastern conformation** is very close to the sloping pasterns seen in breeds such as the German Shepherd Dog.

Health of a dog's organs of locomotion is often reflected in the conformation of the limbs. Recognition of variations in limb conformation is useful not only for judging dog shows but also for assessing the potential for performance in athletic events such as field trials and racing.

A.

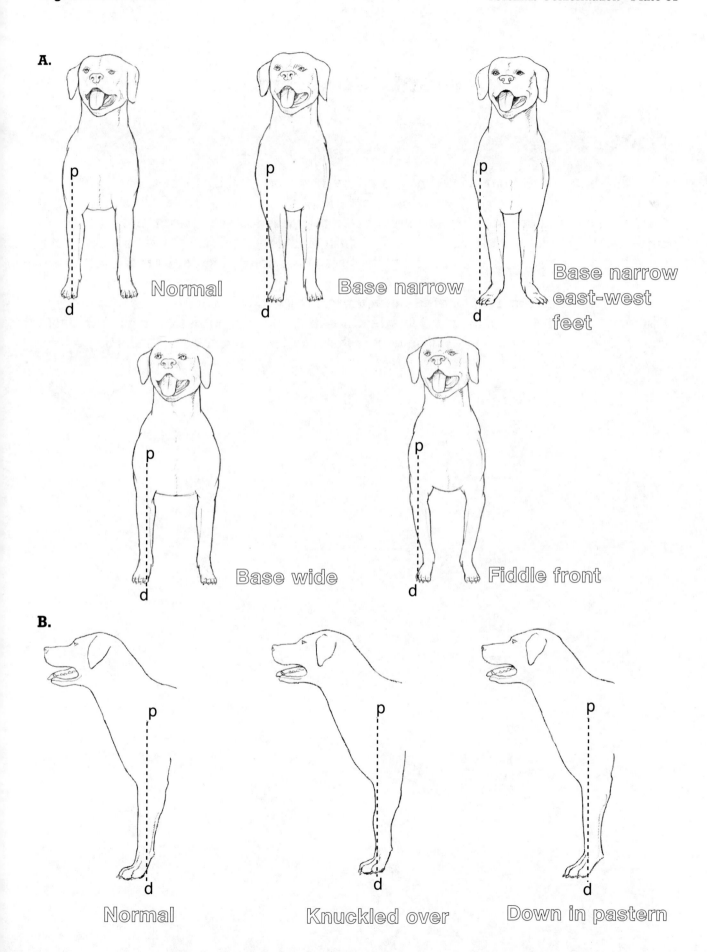

Normal

Base narrow

Base narrow
east-west
feet

Base wide

Fiddle front

B.

Normal

Knuckled over

Down in pastern

Hindlimb Conformation

PLATE 38

Color the dashed lines from **p** (proximal) to **d** (distal) on each of the drawings.

Caudally, a line dropped from the ischiadic tuber to the ground bisects a **normal hindlimb**. The **cow-hocked conformation** places excessive strain on the medial aspect of each hock. Strain is placed on the lateral and plantar aspects of the hock in the **bandy leg conformation**.

In a lateral view of **normal angulated hindquarters**, a line dropped from the ischiatic tuber falls to the ground ahead of the toes. In **straight stifles**, the line touches the toes. The latter conformation places strain on the movement of the patella in the trochlea of the femur.

Caudal views:

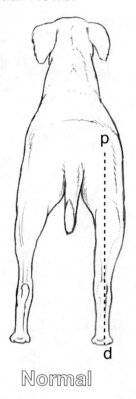

Normal

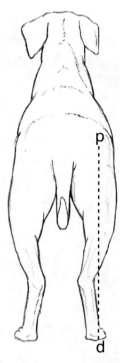

Cow-hocked

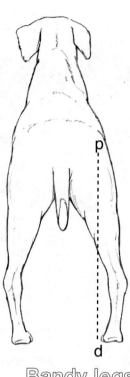

Bandy legs

Lateral views:

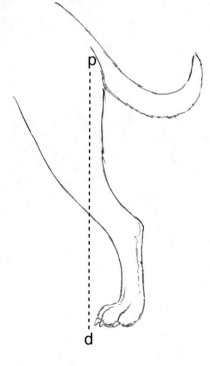

Normal

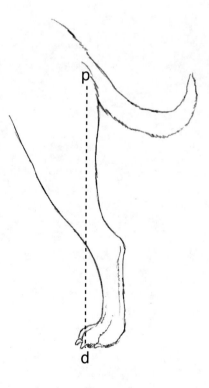

Straight stifles

The Dog's Head

The Skull and Associated Bones

PLATE 39

Figure 1. Lateral view of skull, mandible, and hyoid apparatus.
Figure 2. Dorsal view of skull.

Color the names and the bones that they label.
Underline the following parts of bones and identify them on the drawings:

1. **External occipital protuberance**
2. **Nuchal crest**
3. **Occipital condyle**
4. **Jugular process**
5. **Tympanic bulla**
6. **Ext. acoustic meatus**
7. **Zygomatic arch**
8. **Coronoid process** (of mandible)

9. **Temporomandibular joint**
10. **Angular process**
11. **Mandibular foramen** (on medial side)
12. **Mental foramina**
13. **Infraorbital foramen**
14. **Sagittal crest**
15. **Zygomatic process**
16. **Palatine fissure**

Since sutures are fibrous joints that ossify with age, junctions between most bones of the skull become indistinct.

The inner end of the **external acoustic meatus** is covered by the eardrum (tympanic membrane). The **tympanic bulla** covers the middle ear, and the inner ear is contained within the petrous part of the **temporal bone**.

The **hyoid apparatus** consists of nine small bones and two cartilages that attach to the skull. This arrangement of bones joins the skull to the thyroid cartilage of the larynx and the base of the tongue in which the unpaired basihyoid bone is embedded.

Figure 1

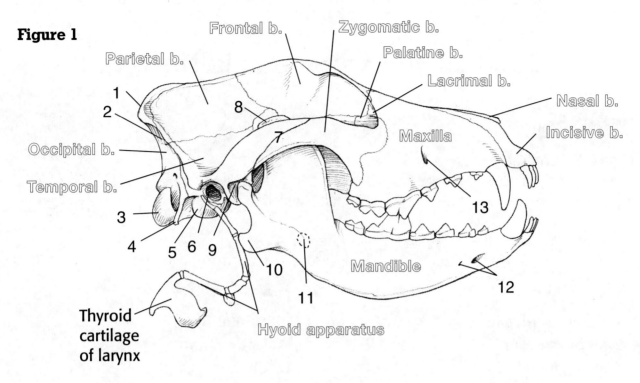

Parietal b.
Frontal b.
Zygomatic b.
Palatine b.
Lacrimal b.
Nasal b.
Incisive b.
Maxilla
Occipital b.
Temporal b.
Mandible
Thyroid cartilage of larynx
Hyoid apparatus

1
2
8
7
3
4
5
6
9
10
11
12
13

Figure 2

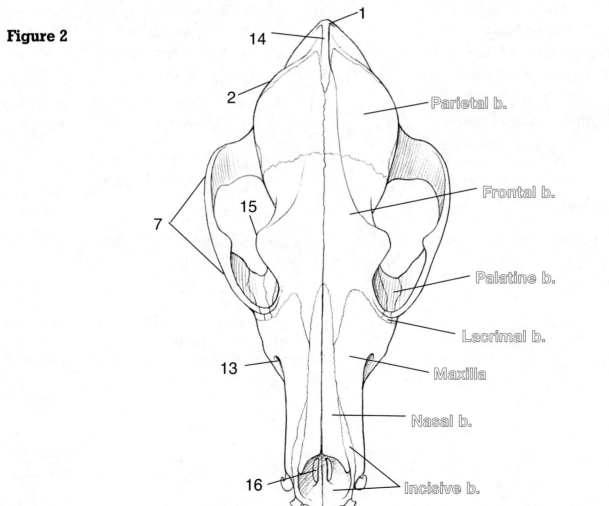

1
14
2
Parietal b.
7
15
Frontal b.
Palatine b.
Lacrimal b.
13
Maxilla
Nasal b.
16
Incisive b.

Cavities and Openings in the Skull

PLATE 40

Figure 1. Ventrolateral view of skull.
Figure 2. Sagittal (parallel to median plane) section (cut) of skull to the left of the nasal septum.
Figure 3. Outline of paranasal sinuses from the exterior.

Color the names and the bones and cavities they label.
Underline the following structures and openings and identify them by the numbers on the drawings:

1. **Foramen magnum**
2. **Occipital condyle**
3. **Hypoglossal canal**
4. **Tympano-occipital fissure**
5. **Tympanic bulla**
6. **Stylomastoid foramen**
7. **Retroarticular foramen**
8. **Oval foramen**
9. **Rostral alar foramen**
10. **Orbital fissure**
11. **Optic canal**
12. **Choana**
13. **Palatine fissure**
14. **Osseous tentorium**
15. **Int. acoustic meatus**
16. **Condyloid canal**
17. **Cribriform plate**
18. **Nasal cavity**

Blood vessels and cranial nerves pass through the foramina (plural of foramen), canals and fissures in the skull. The spinal cord and blood vessels leave the **cranial cavity** through the **foramen magnum**.

A **choana** is the caudal opening of one half of the **nasal cavity**. Left and right halves (nasal fossae) of this cavity are separated by the **nasal septum**, a bony, cartilaginous, and membranous partition.

Paranasal sinuses are mucous membrane-lined cavities that open into the **nasal cavity** on each side. The **maxillary recess** is not a true sinus because it is not fully enclosed by the maxilla. A lateral nasal gland is located in the mucous membrane of the maxillary recess. Its duct opens into the nasal vestibule just behind the nostril (see Plate 43).

Figure 1

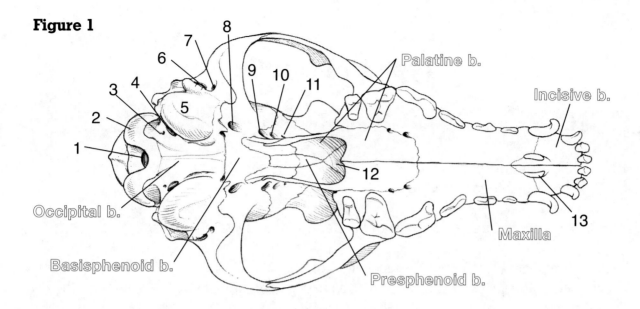

8
7
6
3 4
2
5
1
9 10 11

Palatine b.

Incisive b.

12

Occipital b.

13

Basisphenoid b.

Presphenoid b.

Maxilla

Figure 2

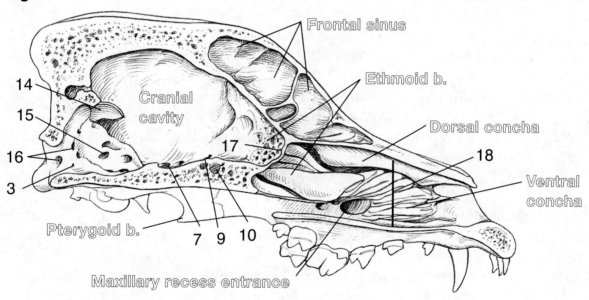

Frontal sinus

Ethmoid b.

14

Cranial cavity

Dorsal concha

15

16

17

18

3

Ventral concha

Pterygoid b.

7 9 10

Maxillary recess entrance

Figure 3

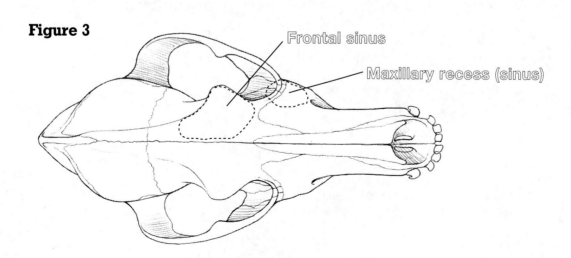

Frontal sinus

Maxillary recess (sinus)

Types of Skulls

PLATE 41

The large diversity in the shapes of dogs' heads has been used as a basis for classifying the various breeds of dogs.

Color the names of the three skull types and the arrows indicating the **stops**.

A stop is a dorsoventral step-down at the junction of the frontal bones with the two maxillae and two nasal bones. This junction and the size and shape of the frontal sinuses determine the extent of the stop.

A **dolichocephalic skull** forms the basis of the long, narrow head of the Greyhound, Borzoi and Collie. The flat stop on a head with a dolichocephalic skull is difficult to see. Notice that the upper incisor teeth (most rostral teeth) slightly overlap the lower incisors, forming a so-called scissors bite. There is a tendency for a marked overshot bite or parrot mouth in this type of skull.

The **mesaticephalic skull** is the commonest skull type, occurring in various canine heads. A smooth, sloping or even a decided stop may be seen on a head with a mesaticephalic skull. Frontal bones are elevated in breeds such as the Pointer and Newfoundland, giving the head a decided stop. Dorsal curving of the nasal bones and the maxillae to their junction with the frontal bones eliminates a stop in the heads of the Bedlington Terrier and the Bull Terrier.

A **brachycephalic skull** is typical of short-faced breeds such as the English Bulldog, Pekingnese, Pug and Boston Terrier. Extreme, deep stops occur on their heads. Notice that the lower incisor teeth extend slightly rostral to the upper incisors in this specimen. There is a tendency for a marked undershot bite in these breeds, a condition known as prognathism. Other defects observed in some brachycephalic heads are wry mouth, in which the mandible is twisted to one side, and lolling tongue, a tongue too long to be retained within the mouth.

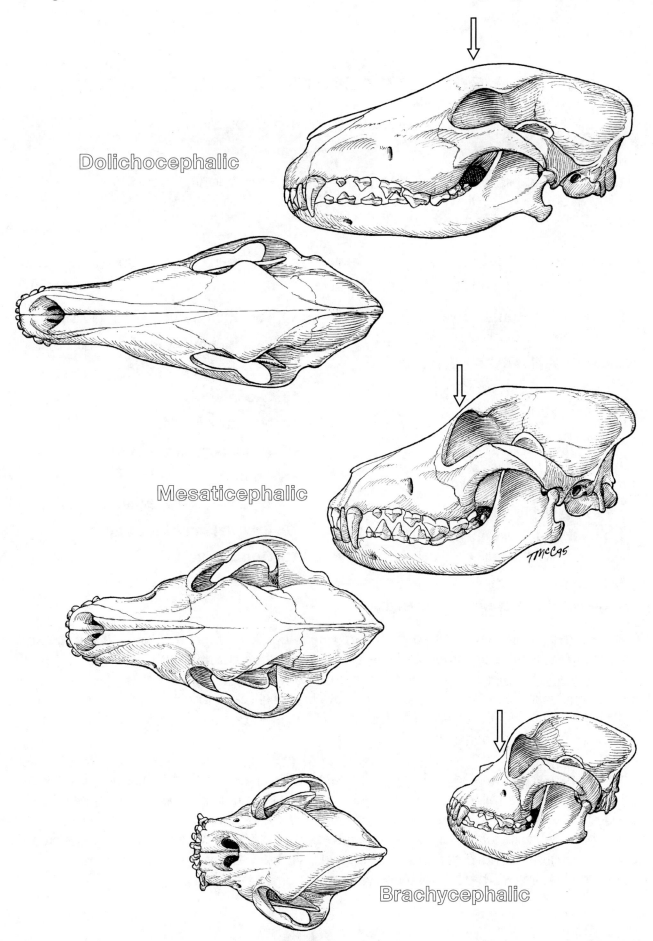

Dolichocephalic

Mesaticephalic

Brachycephalic

The Eye and Accessory Ocular Structures

PLATE 42

Figure 1. The visible eye and accessory structures. Deeper structures outlined.
Figure 2. Course of the flow of tears. Trace the structures involved.
Figure 3. Sagittal section of the eye.

Underline each **boldfaced term** below in a different color. Then color the structure labeled on the drawing in the same color.

1. Reflection of **conjunctiva** – lining of eyelids and anterior eye. Color dotted line.

2. **Lacrimal gland** – secretes tears.

3. **Lateral commissure** – junction of palpebrae (L., eyelids).

4. **Scelera** – fibrous "white of eye".

5. **Iris** – Looking through cornea, C. Muscles control size of pupil.

6. **Pupil** – opening in 5.

7. **Tarsal gland openings** – dots. Lower palpebra pulled down.

8. **Third eyelid** – cartilage outlined.

9. **Gland of 3rd eyelid** – secretes tears.

10. **Lacrimal caruncle** – an elevation

11. **Lacrimal punctum** – opening in palpebra

12. **Lacrimal canaliculi**

13. **Lacrimal sac**

14. **Nasolacrimal duct**

15. **Nasal punctum of 14**

16. **Choroid** – vascular layer.

17. **Tapetum** – reflective region In the choroid.

18. **External muscles of eye**

19. **Optic nerve**

20. **Blood vessels to retina**

Color the path of light (arrow) through the transparent parts of the eye: **cornea (C), anterior chamber (A), posterior chamber (P), lens (L), vitreous chamber (V), and retina (R).** Watery aqueous humor fills the anterior and posterior chambers; the jelly-like vitreous body fills the vitreous chamber. The cornea and lens both bend light rays, focusing them on the retina. Light hitting photoreceptive cells in the retina starts a series of nerve impulses in other cells carried to the brain by nerve fibers in the optic nerve.

Dogs are partially color blind, seeing only blue and yellow. They can see under low light levels due to the reflective **tapetum** increasing the function of the retina. A bright light directed into the dog's eye is reflected by the tapetum, causing the eye to shine. The color of tapetal reflection varies with coat color, e.g., green in black Labrador Retrievers,.yellow in buff-colored Cocker Spaniels. The reflection is blue in puppies, since the eye is not fully developed until six to eight months of age. The eyes of a dog with an abnormal tapetum will reflect red.

Figure 1

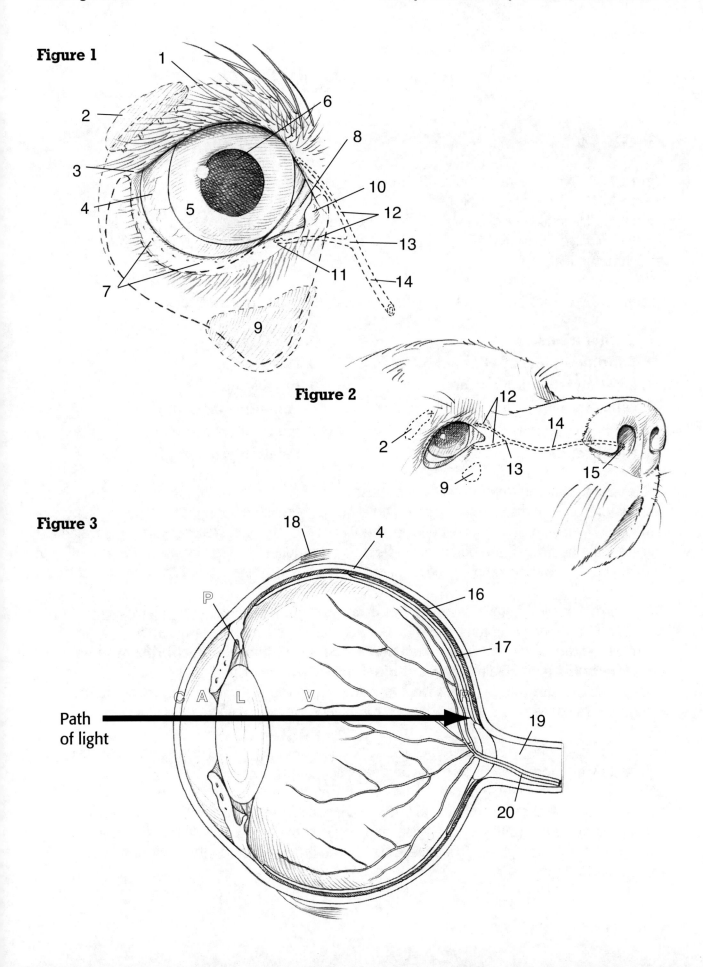

Figure 2

Figure 3

Path
of light

The Dog's Nose

PLATE 43

Figure 1. A. Normal external nose. B. Extreme brachycephalic variation.
Figure 2. Nasal cartilages. Color each of the three cartilages a different color.
Figure 3. Distribution of olfactory nerves in the mucous membrane of the nasal septum and ethmoturbinates. Sagittal view. Part of the bony nasal septum removed to expose the left ethmoturbinates.

Underline the names below and color the names on the plate different colors.

1. **Ethmoturbinates**
2. **Cribriform plate of ethmoid b.**
3. **Right olfactory bulb of brain**
4. **Olfactory nerve fibers**
5. **Ethmoidal nerve**
6. **Nasal septum**
7. **Nasal cartilages**
8. **Nasal bone**
9. **Incisive duct**
10. **Vomeronasal organ**
11. **Vomeronasal nerves**
12. **Palatine process of maxilla**

Complicated nasal cartilages and attached muscles change the shape of the nostrils. There are no hairs or glands in the normally pigmented skin. The "healthy" cool nose is kept moist by lacrimal and lateral nasal gland secretions (see Plate 66). These secretions humidify inhaled air and dissipate heat when the dog pants. The pattern of ridges in the thick skin here is unique to individual dogs. Thus, nose prints are similar to human fingerprints. Color the names.

Olfactory mucous membrane covers half of **ethmoturbinates** of the ethmoidal labyrinth, the caudal half of the nasal septum, and much of the walls of the caudal nasal cavity. Substances in the mucus stimulate olfactory cells. Their **nerve fibers** pass through the **cribriform plate** to the **olfactory bulbs** of the brain. The **ethmoidal nerve** senses irritation and causes sneezing. A dog's sense of smell (olfaction) is several hundred times more sensitive than that of humans. A Bloodhound's olfaction is a thousand times more sensitive.

Odors of pheromones produced by related individuals or during heat (estrus) in females are detected by olfactory neurons in each vomeronasal organ (organ of Jacobsen). Supported by a scroll of cartilage, this tubule of olfactory mucous membrane opens into an **incisive duct** which opens into the nasal cavity and next to the incisive papilla in the oral cavity. In the flehmen response in a male dog, the tongue licks rapidly against the hard palate, the upper lips curl and the incisor teeth part slightly. This forces pheromone-bearing mucus into the incisive ducts and vomeronasal organs.

Figure 1

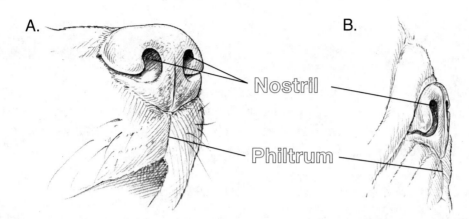

A. B.

Nostril

Philtrum

Figure 2

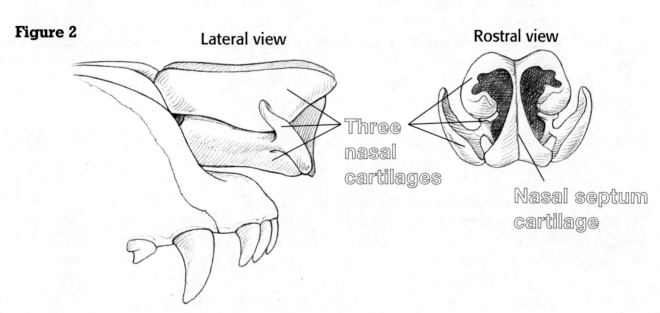

Lateral view Rostral view

Three
nasal
cartilages

Nasal septum
cartilage

Figure 3

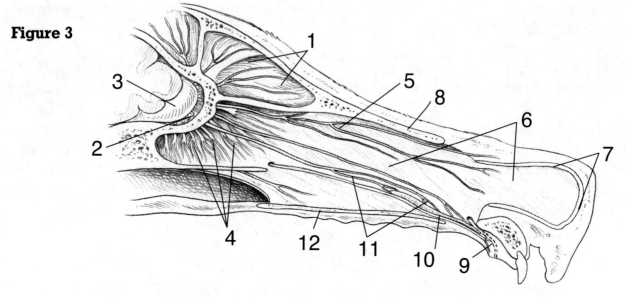

The Dog's Ear

PLATE 44

Figure 1. External ear. Drawing of a dissection exposing the ear canal.
Figure 2. Middle ear and inner ear. Schematic drawing of the temporal bone showing the auditory ossicles (little ear bones – **malleus**, **incus** and **stapes**) of the middle ear and the **cochlea**, **semicircular canals**, **utricle** and **saccule** of the inner ear.

Color the names on the drawings and color the structures where appropriate.

The **pinna's auricular cartilage** assumes many shapes and sizes in different breeds of dogs. Auricular (ear) muscles act independently on each side of the head, directing the pinna toward the sound. Notice the bend between the **vertical ear canal** and the **horizontal ear canal**. Skin lining the ear canal contains many apocrine tubular and sebaceous glands. Their combined secretions forms the dry, brownish cerumen (ear wax). When the ear canal is inflamed by ear mites or an infection, the secretion increases and is more liquid.

An **auditory tube** extends from the nasopharynx to the middle ear, serving to equalize pressure on each side of the eardrum.

Sound waves in the ear canal vibrate the **eardrum**. The **malleus** (partly embedded in the eardrum) **incus** and **stapes** gear down the vibrations and transmit them to a liquid in the inner ear. These vibrations move membranes in the **cochlea** that stimulate hair cells, producing nerve impulses carried to the brain by the vestibulocochlear nerve. The dog's cochlea is larger than man's. The dog's hearing is far more sensitive than that of man. Sound wave frequency limits in man are 20 to 20,000 cycles per second. In dogs, the upper limit is around 40,000 cycles per second. Frequencies emitted by a dog whistle are above the upper limit of human hearing but below a dog's upper limit.

Sometimes a pup of a white breed, e.g., a Dalmatian or a pup with a predominantly white head is born deaf. Hearing loss is common in old dogs. A dog's hearing can be accurately tested.

Three **semicircular ducts** (within bony canals) situated at approximately 90 degrees to one another contain a liquid that stimulates a sensory region in each canal. These regions are stimulated by changes in the position of the head. Sensory regions in the **utricle** and **saccule** are stimulated by positive or negative linear acceleration. Nerve impulses from these sensory regions in the vestibule of the inner ear are carried to the brain by the vestibulocochlear nerve.

Figure 1

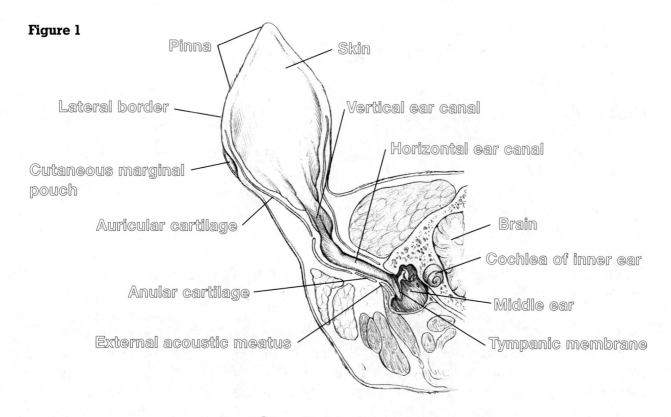

Pinna

Skin

Lateral border

Vertical ear canal

Horizontal ear canal

Cutaneous marginal pouch

Auricular cartilage

Brain

Cochlea of inner ear

Anular cartilage

Middle ear

External acoustic meatus

Tympanic membrane

Figure 2

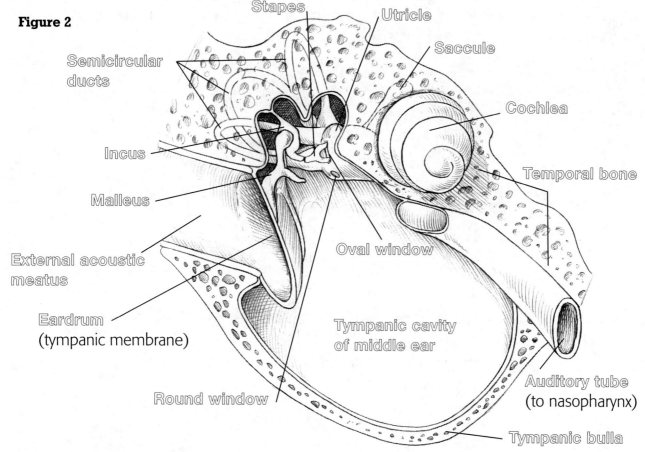

Stapes

Utricle

Saccule

Semicircular ducts

Cochlea

Incus

Temporal bone

Malleus

External acoustic meatus

Oval window

Eardrum
(tympanic membrane)

Tympanic cavity
of middle ear

Round window

Auditory tube
(to nasopharynx)

Tympanic bulla

External Ear Types

PLATE 45

The auricular cartilage of the pinna assumes many shapes and sizes in different breeds of dogs. There are three basic ear types: **erect (pricked) ears, semi-erect (semipricked) ears,** and **pendulous (drop) ears**. The position and carriage of the external ears is influenced by the shape of the head and the tension exerted by the auricular muscles attached to the cartilage. The amount of hair also adds to the shape and carriage of the ear.

On the drawings of selected external ear types, color each name in a different color and color the indicated ears the same color.

Otitis externa is inflammation of the external ear, mainly the ear canal. The cause of otitis externa varies. Several kinds of bacteria, molds, and yeasts that may even be found in healthy ears cause disease. Ear mites, foreign bodies, and trauma to the ear canal are other causes of inflammation. Grass and seeds are foreign bodies that are commonly found in the ear canal, when the heads of the plants ripen. Whereas otitis externa can occur in all types of ears, breeds with long hair and pendulous (drop) ears are more frequently affected. The tips of erect ears are subject to inflammation caused by fly bites.

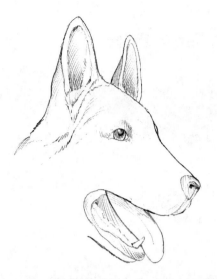

Erect (pricked) ears

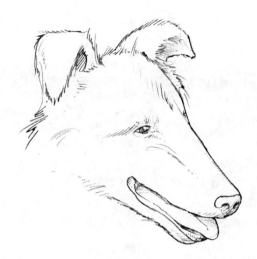

Semi-erect (semi-pricked) ears

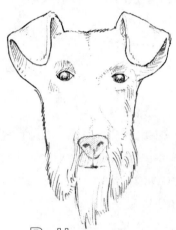

Button ears

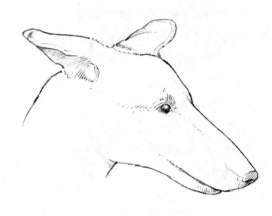

Flying ears

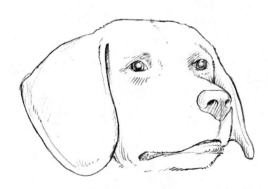

Pendulous (drop) ears

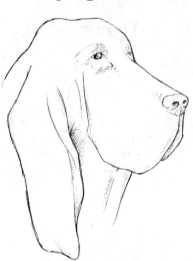

Pendulous, folded and curled ears

Lateral Structures of the Head

PLATE 46

Figure 1. Major superficial muscles. Platysma and superficial cervical sphincter muscles removed.
Figure 2. Superficial veins and nerves. Salivary glands.

Underline each **boldfaced name** in color. Then locate and color the structure
labeled on the drawings in the same color. Use blue for veins; yellow for nerves.
m. = muscle; v. = vein; n. = nerve .

1. **Mental m.**
2. **Oral orbicular m.** (cut)
3. **Canine m.**
4. **Maxillary lip levator m.**
5. **Nasolabial levator m.** (cut)
6. **Ocular orbicular m.**
7. **Zygomatic m.**
8. **Frontal m.**
9. **Zygomaticoauricular m.**
10. **Cervicoauricular muscles**
11. **Temporal m.**
12. **Parotid gland**
13. **Mandibular gland**
14. **External jugular v.**
15. **Parotidoauricular m.**

16. **Mandibular lymph nodes**
17. **Masseter m.**
18. **Deep sphincter m. of neck**
19. **Buccinator m.**
20. **Ocular angular v.**
21. **Dorsal buccal branch of facial n.**
22. **Facial v.**
23. **Parotid duct**
24. **Ventral buccal branch of facial n.**
25. **Second cervical n.**
26. **Great auricular n.**
27. **Maxillary v.**
28. **Linguofacial v.**
29. **Buccal salivary gland**
30. **Buccal lymph node**

Figure 1

Figure 2

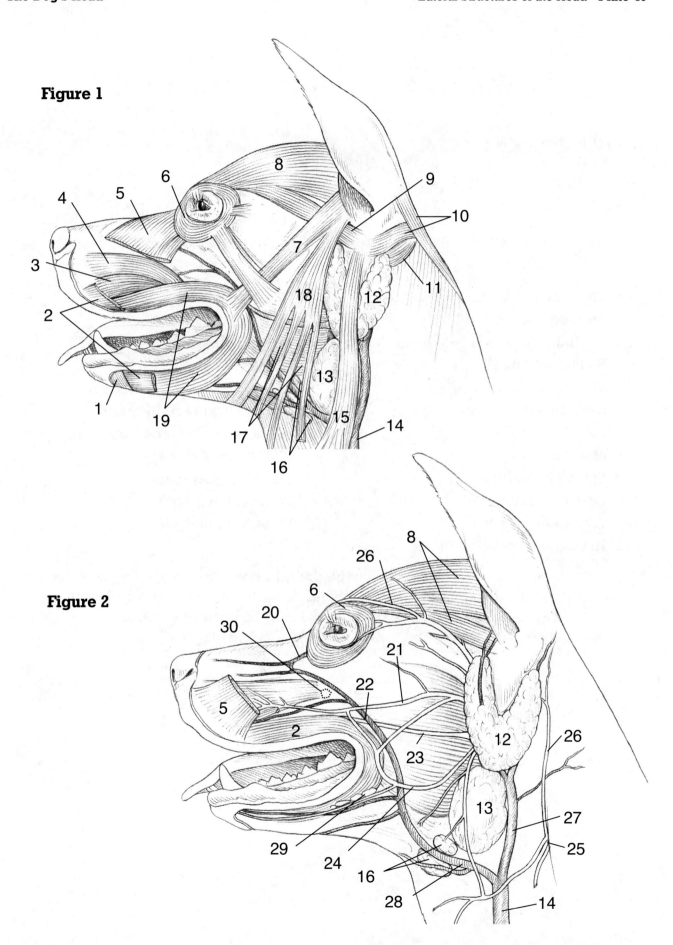

Ventral Structures of the Head

PLATE 47

Figure 1. Ventral superficial muscles of the head. m. = muscle.
Figure 2. Deeper dissection of ventral aspect of the head.

Underline each **boldfaced name** in a different color. Then locate and color the organ labeled on the drawings in the same color.

1. **Sternocephalic m.**
2. **Sternohyoid m.**
3. **Medial retropharyngeal lymph node**
4. **Basihyoid bone**
5. **Stylohyoid m.**
6. **Digastric m.**
7. **Masseter m.**
8. **Mylohyoid m.**
9. **Sternothyroid m.**
10. **First cervical nerve**
11. **Cranial laryngeal nerve**
12. **Hypoglossal nerve**

13. **Lingual artery**
14. **Hyoglossal m.**
15. **Styloglossal m.**
16. **Geniohyoid m.**
17. **Genioglossal m.**
18. **Common carotid artery**
19. **Vagosympathetic trunk**
20. **Mandibular gland**
21. **Sublingual gland**
22. **Major sublingual duct**
23. **Mandibular duct**

Of special significance in Figure 2 are the **hypoglossal nerve**, the motor supply to the muscles of the tongue, the **lingual artery**, and the **mandibular** and **sublingual glands** and their ducts. The **vagosympathetic nerve trunk** (along side the **common carotid artery**) carries autonomic nerve fibers to and from the head. (Also see Plate 80.)

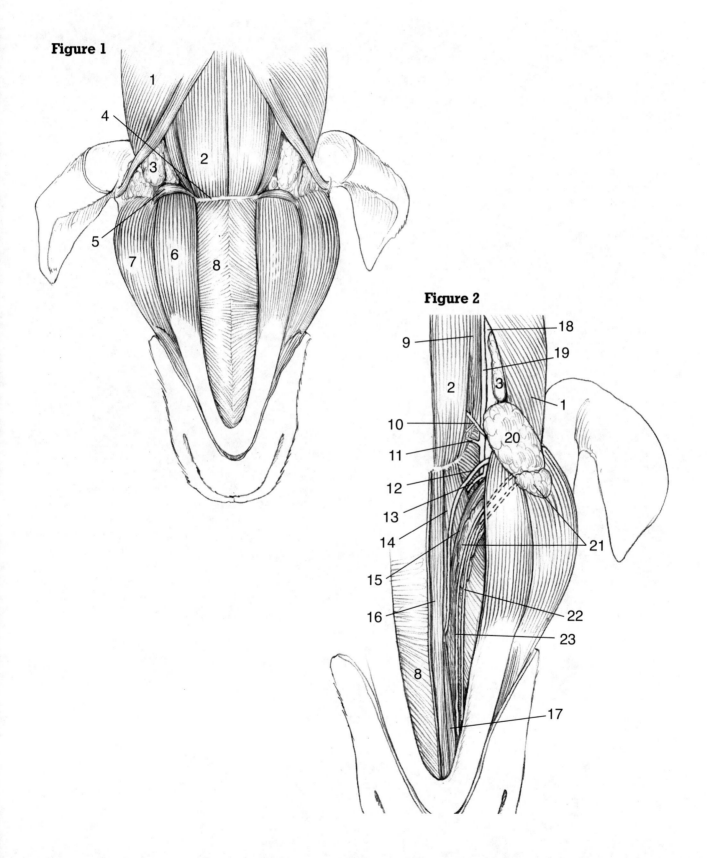

Figure 1

1

4

3

2

5

7

6

8

Figure 2

9

18

19

2

3

1

10

20

11

12

13

14

21

15

16

22

23

8

17

Digestive System

The Dog's Teeth

PLATE 48

Figure 1. The permanent teeth in a mesaticephalic skull.

Underline the names and abbreviations of the teeth listed below in different colors and color the teeth as they are labeled on the drawing. The word, tooth, is usually dropped when referring to specific teeth.

I1 **First incisor tooth**
I2 **Second incisor tooth**
I3 **Third incisor tooth**
 C **Canine tooth**
P1 **First premolar tooth**
P2 **Second premolar tooth**

P3 **Third premolar tooth**
P4 **Fourth premolar tooth**
M1 **First molar tooth**
M2 **Second molar tooth**
M3 **Third molar tooth**

The <u>dental</u> <u>formula</u> for the <u>permanent</u> <u>teeth</u> is **2(I3/3 C1/1 P4/4 M2/3) = 42**

Notice the two large **carnassial (sectorial) teeth** – the upper fourth premolar and the lower first molar. The teeth of the upper dental arch are lateral to those in the lower dental arch. The lower canine tooth bites rostral to the upper canine. The incisor and canine teeth are used for grasping; the carnassial teeth and the rest of the premolars are shearing teeth; the distal part of the lower first molar and the remaining molars are used for grinding.

The usual dental formula for the <u>deciduous</u> <u>teeth</u> is **2(Di3/3 Dc1/1 Dp3/3) = 28** The occasional presence of deciduous upper first molar teeth and the regular occurrence of deciduous lower first molars has been reported in certain breeds of dogs, making the dental formula **2(Di3/3 Dc1l1 Dp3/3 Dm(1)/1 = 30 or 32**

Figure 2. Longitudinal section through a simple tooth.

On the drawing, underline the names and the structures labeled in different colors.

<u>Periodontal</u> (around the tooth) <u>disease</u> is the most common disease of dogs. <u>Tooth</u> <u>fracture</u> is the second most common dental problem. Because of their overlapping alignment, **carnassial teeth** are the most likely to be affected. Soft, light-colored <u>plaque</u> on the tooth and **gingiva** is composed of food particles, bacteria, and deposits of saliva. Minerals in saliva will harden plaque into **tartar (calculus)** that will expand in the **gingival groove**, irritating the gum and causing <u>gingivitis</u> (inflammation of the gums). This leads to <u>periodontitis</u>. Bacteria multiply, causing bleeding and tissue loss, destruction of the **periodontal ligament** and loosening of the tooth. Inflammation spreads to **alveolar bone**, causing bone loss and, eventually, loss of the tooth.

<u>Dental</u> <u>caries</u> (tooth decay) is rare in dogs.

Figure 1

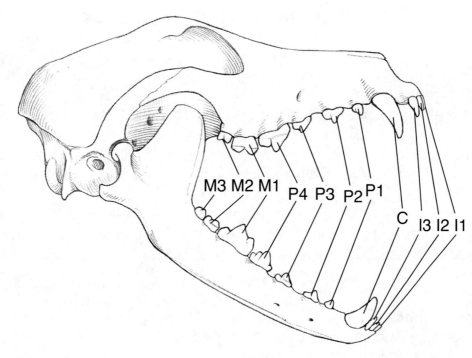

M3 M2 M1   P4 P3 P2 P1

C   I3 I2 I1

Figure 2

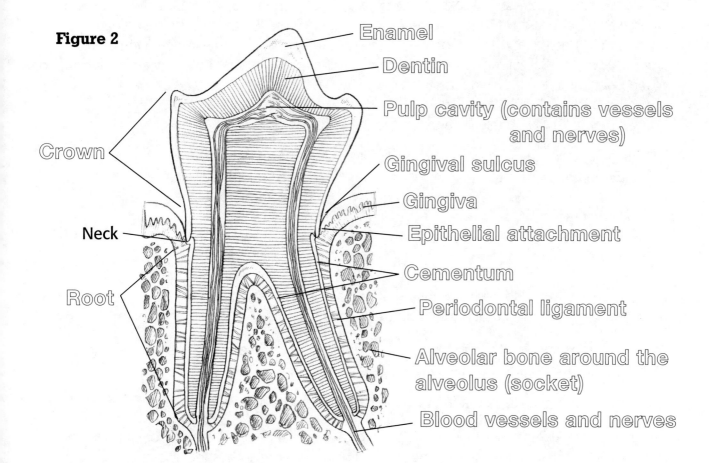

Enamel

Dentin

Pulp cavity (contains vessels and nerves)

Gingival sulcus

Gingiva

Epithelial attachment

Cementum

Periodontal ligament

Alveolar bone around the alveolus (socket)

Blood vessels and nerves

Crown

Neck

Root

Dental Variations in Dogs

PLATE 49

Figure 1. Comparison of upper teeth in a mesaticephalic head, A, and a brachycephalic head, B.

Identify and label the teeth in different colors, using the abbreviations (I1, I2, etc.) presented in Plate 48. Notice crowding of the teeth and rotation of the premolars in the brachycephalic head.

In extreme brachycephalic heads, <u>cheek</u> <u>teeth</u> (premolars and molars) can be missing at each end of the dental arcade. In dolichocephalic breeds, the cheek teeth are farther apart. In all breeds, extra teeth are occasionally present. The most common extra teeth are the incisors and premolars.

Dental Eruption Times
Different references vary in the times given for eruption of the deciduous and permanent teeth. In general, deciduous canine teeth erupt between 3 and 5 weeks of age followed by the deciduous incisors at 4 to 6 weeks. Deciduous premolars (Dp2, 3, 4) erupt between 5 and 6 weeks with Dp4 possibly erupting a week or two later. There is no Dp1; the permanent first premolar (P1) erupts at 4 to 5 months. When present, deciduous molar teeth would erupt at around 8 weeks. Sometimes a deciduous tooth, especially a canine tooth, remains after eruption of the permanent tooth. Such persistent deciduous teeth should be extracted.

A dog's permanent teeth usually erupt at the following ages:

I1 3-5 months   P3 5-6 months
I2 3-5 months   P4 4-5 months
I3 4-5 months   M1 5-6 months
 C 5-7 months   M2 5-6 months
P1 4-5 months   M3 6-7 months
P2 5-6 months

A dog is generally said to be <u>full-mouthed</u> at 6 to 7 months. The teeth of large dogs, which have a shorter life span than smaller dogs, erupt earlier.

Figure 2. Appearance of wear changes at different ages. Notice the sequential wearing down of **cusps** (small points), first on the lower incisors.

Color incisor and and canine teeth at each age a different color.

Aging dogs by wear on their teeth is not very reliable. The drawings here are for large dogs with mesaticephalic heads. Small dogs and dogs wirh overshot or undershot jaws cannot be aged satisfactorily using this method.

Figure 1

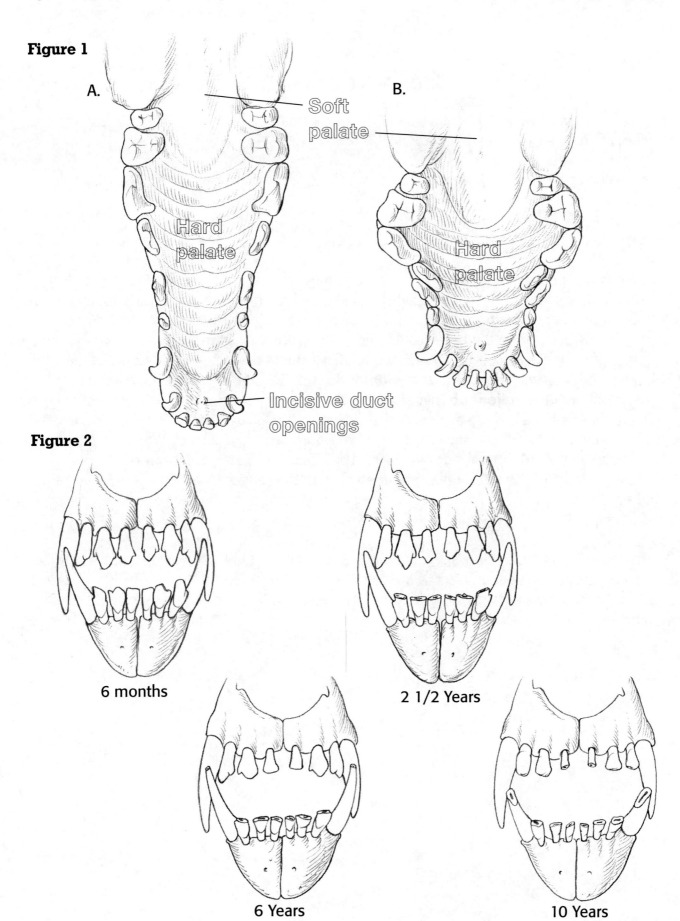

A.   B.

Soft palate

Hard palate   Hard palate

Incisive duct openings

Figure 2

6 months   2 1/2 Years

6 Years   10 Years

Salivary Glands

PLATE 50

Dissection of a dog's head exposing the main salivary glands and their ducts. The mandible has been removed.

Color the names on the drawing in different colors and color the labeled organs the same colors.

The **parotid duct** (cut near its origin in this drawing) crosses the masseter muscle (see Plate 46) and opens into the vestibule (space between the lips and cheeks, and the teeth and gums) opposite the upper fourth premolar tooth. Occasionally, a small accessory parotid gland is present , its duct joining the large parotid duct. The **zygomatic gland** lies just under the orbit. One large and three or four small **zygomatic gland ducts** open into the vestibule caudal to the opening of the parotid duct. The **mandibular duct** crosses the **digastric muscle** and then runs along with the **major sublingual duct** from the **monostomatic** (having one opening) part of the sublingual gland. The two ducts pass between the genioglossal and mylohyoid muscles and are then enclosed by a sublingual fold of mucous membrane as they extend to their openings on the **sublingual papilla**. Several tiny ducts from the **polystomatic** (having several openings) **part of the sublingual gland** empty into the ventrocaudal vestibule. Several small buccal glands secrete onto the mucous membrane of the cheek. The tongue also contains salivary glands.

The salivary glands' secretion, saliva, moistens and lubricates food for chewing and swallowing. In the dog, evaporation of abundant saliva, particularly on the surface of the tongue, has a cooling effect on the body similar to the evaporation of sweat in man. The dog's sweat glands rarely produce a liquid sweat.

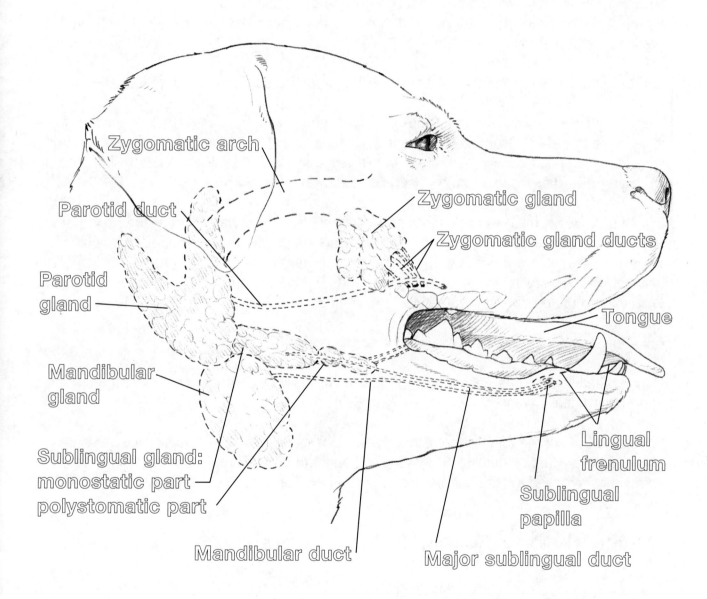

Zygomatic arch

Parotid duct

Zygomatic gland

Zygomatic gland ducts

Parotid gland

Tongue

Mandibular gland

Sublingual gland:
monostatic part
polystomatic part

Lingual frenulum

Sublingual papilla

Mandibular duct

Major sublingual duct

Oral Cavity, Tongue, Pharynx, and Esophagus

PLATE 51

Figure 1. Right lateral view of a sagittal section of a dog's head.
Figure 2. Dorsal view of the tongue and dissected laryngopharynx, trachea, and esophagus.
Figure 3. A puppy's tongue.

Color each label in a different color and, where appropriate, color the structure indicated.

The **pharynx** is a musculomembranous chamber common to the digestive and respiratory tracts. Its three parts are: 1) **Oropharynx** – ventral to the soft palate, 2) **nasopharynx** – dorsal to the soft palate, extending caudad from the choanae (exits from the nasal fossa on each side), 3) **laryngopharynx** - dorsal to the larynx and leading into the **esophagus**.

During swallowing, muscles raise the **tongue**, pressing food and water against the **hard palate**. The **soft palate** is elevated. The root of the tongue moves caudad and dorsad in a boltlike manner, pushing the **epiglottis** partially over the **laryngeal entrance**. The rima glottidis (space between the vocal folds) in the larynx is narrowed. Pressure by pharyngeal muscles forces food or water into the esophagus where automatic contractions carry food through to the stomach.

Color the dashed line indicating the movement of food or water.

During breathing, the free edge of the soft palate is usually (but not always) under the epiglottis, and the laryngeal entrance is open (see Plate 67).

Within the apex of the tongue, the rodlike **lyssa** consists of adipose tissue, skeletal muscle and some cartilage. In olden times, the lyssa was thought to be the cause of rabies, and it was sometimes removed to cure the disease. What a place for one's hands! Lyssa is also a synonym for rabies.

Vallate, foliate, and **fungiform papillae** contain taste buds, a complex of gustatory (taste) cells, supporting cells and nerve endings.

Conical, filiform, and **marginal papillae** do not contain taste buds.

Marginal papillae on a neonatal (newborn) puppy's tongue assist in suckling. As the diet changes from milk to solid food, marginal papillae regress until they no longer exist.

Figure 1

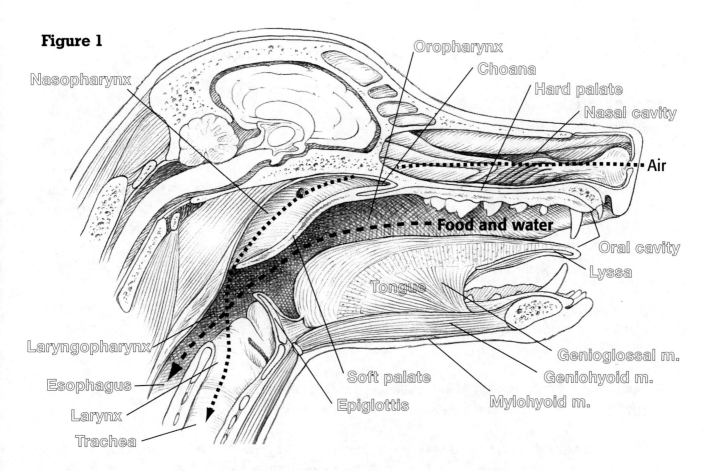

Nasopharynx

Oropharynx

Choana

Hard palate

Nasal cavity

Air

Food and water

Oral cavity

Lyssa

Tongue

Laryngopharynx

Genioglossal m.

Geniohyoid m.

Esophagus

Soft palate

Mylohyoid m.

Larynx

Epiglottis

Trachea

Figure 2

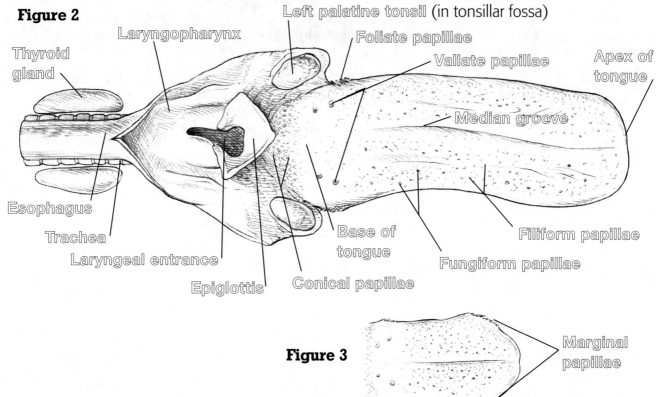

Laryngopharynx

Left palatine tonsil (in tonsillar fossa)

Foliate papillae

Vallate papillae

Apex of tongue

Thyroid gland

Median groove

Esophagus

Trachea

Base of tongue

Filiform papillae

Laryngeal entrance

Fungiform papillae

Epiglottis

Conical papillae

Figure 3

Marginal papillae

Contents of the Abdominal Cavity

PLATE 52

Figure 1. The abdominal wall and the thoracic muscles have been removed in this ventral view. The **greater omentum,** a double fold of peritoneum (serous membrane of the abdominal and pelvic cavities), enfolds the ventral and lateral aspects of the coils of the small intestine. A superficial leaf extends caudad from the surface of the stomach to near the urinary bladder, then turns back as a deep leaf that returns craniad to attach again to the stomach. The collapsed cavity between the two leaves is called the omental bursa. It communicates with the main peritoneal cavity through a small opening.

Notice the long deposits of fat (adipose tissue) that occur along small vessels in the greater omentum. Color the fat yellow. Use light red lines to indicate the rest of the greater omentum, which is transparent in life.

Minor parts of the greater omentum include an extension to the spleen, the gastrosplenic ligament, and a part that encloses some of the left lobe of the pancreas.

As a storage place for fat, large amounts accumulate in the greater omentum in obese dogs. The greater omentum provides a protective function to the immune cells it contains. It assists injured tissues in forming new blood vessels. Once removed, the greater omentum does not regenerate. However, dogs from whom most of the greater omentum has been removed remain healthy.

Figure 2. The greater omentum has been removed, revealing the organs that it covered. Color the names and organs indicated.

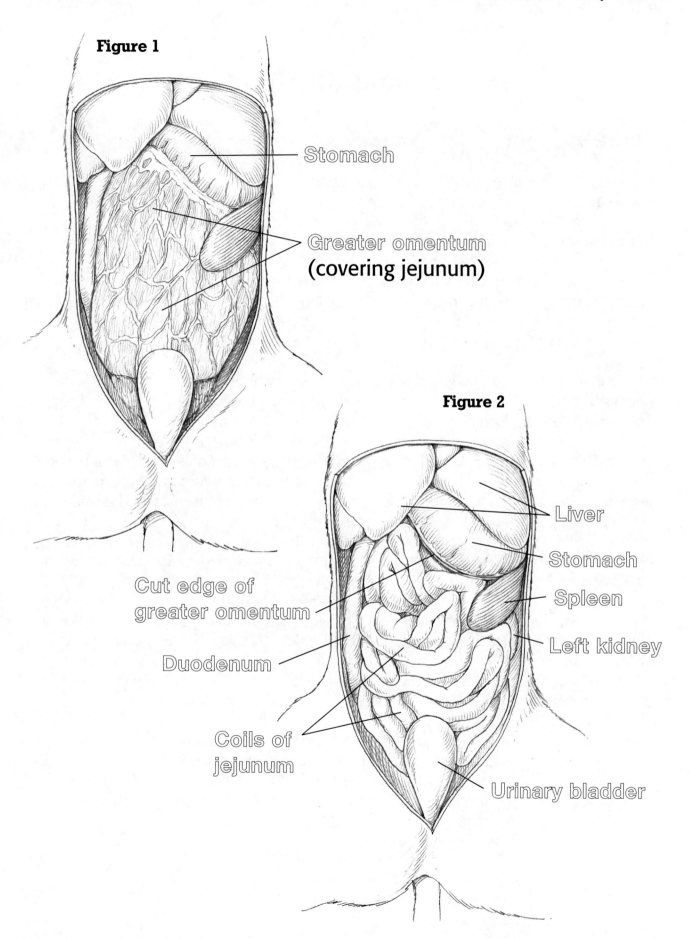

Figure 1

Stomach

Greater omentum
(covering jejunum)

Figure 2

Liver

Stomach

Spleen

Left kidney

Cut edge of
greater omentum

Duodenum

Coils of
jejunum

Urinary bladder

Stomach and Small Intestine

PLATE 53

Figure 1. Ventral view of canine stomach and small intestine (shortened).
Figure 2. Stomach and first part of the duodenum sectioned to expose the lining.

Using different colors, color the names, parts, and regions indicated by the lines.
In Figure 1, the stomach is moderately full. Size and shape of the stomach vary greatly, depending on the amount of feed (or gas) it contains. When empty, it does not touch the abdominal wall. When full, particularly in puppies, it pushes against and distends the abdominal wall. Branches for the celiac artery course along the lesser and greater curvatures. Venous drainage is through branches of the portal vein to the liver.

Glands in the **proper gastric gland region** secrete hydrochloric acid and the enzymes pepsin (digests protein) and rennin (curdles milk). Superficial lining cells of the <u>mucous</u> <u>membrane</u> of the stomach secrete protective <u>mucus</u>.

The small intestine, suspended by the peritoneal <u>mesentery</u>, is 3.5 times the length if the body. The bile duct (from the gall bladder) and the major **pancreatic duct open** on the **major duodenal papilla**; the minor **pancreatic duct** opens on the **minor duodenal papilla**. The intestinal mucous membrane secretes enzymes and mucus. The mucous membrane lining the stomach and the small intestine also produce hormones. <u>Peyer's</u> <u>patches</u>, groups of lymphatic nodules, are prominent in the ileum. Branches from the cranial mesenteric artery supply most of the small intestine.

Gastric dilatation-volvulus (GDV), also called <u>bloat</u>, is a condition in dogs in which <u>dilatation</u> (abnormal distention) leads to <u>volvulus</u> (torsion or twisting), closing the cardia and pylorus and interfering with blood flow. This results in the accumulation of gas, and inflammatory processes follow. GDV occurs most often in large dogs with deep chests. Sucking air into the stomach and overeating contribute to this condition. Surgical correction is usually indicated.

Inflammation of the lining of the stomach (<u>gastritis</u>) and the lining of the small intestine (<u>enteritis</u>) may be caused by different organisms or substances.

<u>Vomiting</u> is a natural function in dogs. To prevent excessive vomiting caused by overeating and excited gulping, provide plenty of water and good food in frequent small amounts. Isolate an excitable dog from others while it is eating.

Figure 1

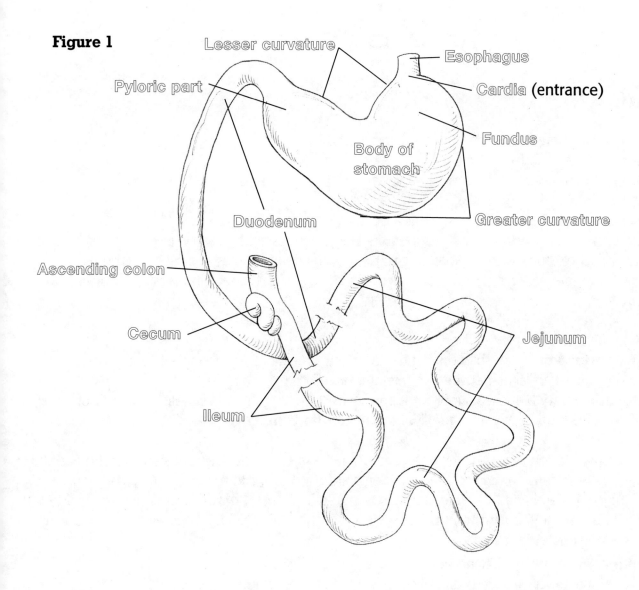

Lesser curvature

Esophagus

Pyloric part

Cardia **(entrance)**

Fundus

Body of
stomach

Duodenum

Greater curvature

Ascending colon

Cecum

Jejunum

Ileum

Figure 2

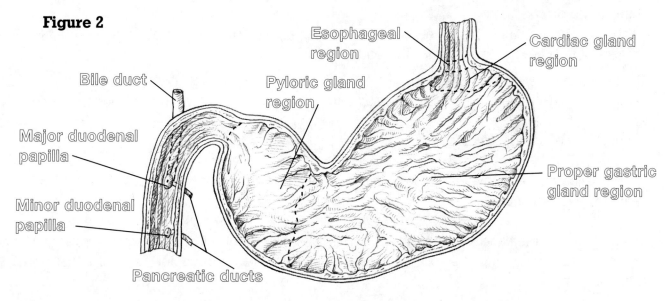

Esophageal
region

Cardiac gland
region

Bile duct

Pyloric gland
region

Major duodenal
papilla

Proper gastric
gland region

Minor duodenal
papilla

Pancreatic ducts

Liver and Pancreas

PLATE 54

Figure 1. Diaphragmatic surface of the canine liver,
Figure 2. Visceral surface of the canine liver.
Figure 3. Ventral view of the canine pancreas and related organs.

Color the names and the structures indicated, using different colors.
Peritoneum covers the **liver**, and four peritoneal ligaments stabilize the liver. The diaphragmatic surface is closely applied to the diaphragm; the visceral surface faces against the abdominal viscera (large internal organs). The stomach, left kidney, and duodenum press firmly against the visceral surface.

Two blood vessels supply the liver:
1) The **portal vein** carries blood from the stomach, small intestine, pancreas, and spleen to the liver's sinusoids, capillaries between sheets of liver cells.
2) **Hepatic artery** branches supply nutrients, especially oxygen, to liver cells. Branches of **hepatic veins** carry blood from the liver to the **caudal vena cava**.

Blood brought to the liver contains absorbed nutrients and also harmful substances. The harmful substances are destroyed by the liver. Nutrients are used to make many essential compounds, including cholesterol and bile. Secreted bile is stored in the **gall bladder** and then transported by the **bile duct** to the **duodenum**. Here it helps to neutralize acid and emulsify fats, breaking up large fat globules into smaller ones.

The **pancreas** is two glands in one:
1) The exocrine part produces digestive enzymes that are carried to the duodenum by **pancreatic ducts**.
2) The endocrine part secretes the hormones glucagon, insulin, and somatostatin into the blood for transport to tissues elsewhere in the body.

These homones are produced by specific cells in masses called pancreatic islets (islets of Langerhans). Glucagon mobilizes blood sugar from the liver; insulin decreases blood sugar; somatostatin inhibits the release of growth hormone from the pituitary gland and reduces contractions of smooth muscle in the intestines and gall bladder.

Inflammation of the liver is termed hepatitis, a disease caused mainly by viruses, although other factors can cause hepatitis. (-itis = inflammation of.)

Inflammation of the pancreas is termed pancreatitis, a disease due to self digestion by its own enzymes. It may be caused by bile duct disease, increased fat in the blood, or trauma (damage) to the abdomen.

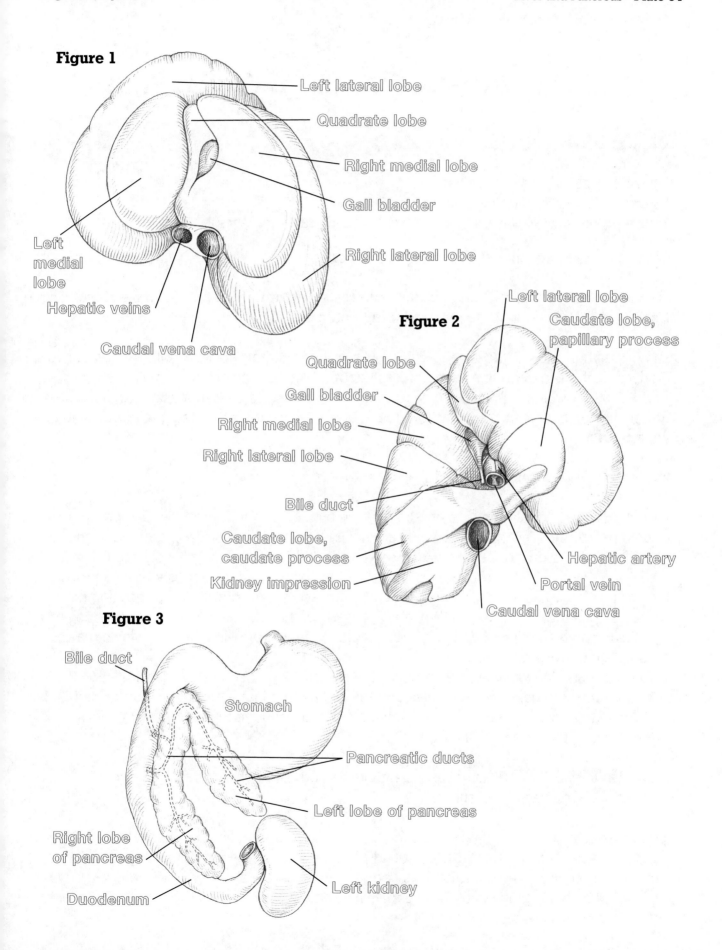

Figure 1

Left lateral lobe

Quadrate lobe

Right medial lobe

Gall bladder

Right lateral lobe

Left medial lobe

Hepatic veins

Caudal vena cava

Figure 2

Left lateral lobe

Caudate lobe, papillary process

Quadrate lobe

Gall bladder

Right medial lobe

Right lateral lobe

Bile duct

Caudate lobe, caudate process

Kidney impression

Hepatic artery

Portal vein

Caudal vena cava

Figure 3

Bile duct

Stomach

Pancreatic ducts

Left lobe of pancreas

Right lobe of pancreas

Left kidney

Duodenum

Large Intestine, Anus, and Anal Sacs

PLATE 55

Figure 1. Isolated large intestine.
Figure 2. Caudal view of the anus of the male dog.
Figure 3. Dorsal view of sectioned rectum, anal canal, and anal sacs.

Color the names, the organs, and the regions indicated.

The large intestine consists of the **cecum, colon,** and **rectum**. The cecum and the **ileum** of the small intestine both empty into the **ascending colon**.

The primary functions of the large intestine are the absorption of water and a few other nutrients, production of mucus, and formation of feces (stool). Like the stomach and small intestine, smooth muscle in the wall of the colon functions in peristalsis, the wave of contraction that moves the contents of these organs toward the anus. Notice the expanded part of the rectum, the **ampulla**.

Inflammation of the colon is termed colitis.

Each **anal sac** is actually a pouch of skin, opening by means of a duct on the **cutaneous zone** of the **anal canal**. The walls of an anal sac contain large, modified sweat glands. The contents of the anal sacs consist of secretions of these glands and sloughed off cells from the lining epidermis. Normally, anal sacs are expressed by the passage of firm stool and from squeezing by the sphincter muscles on either side of each sac. Accumulation of anal sac secretion may be caused by prolonged soft stool or temporary plugging of the anal sac duct. An affected dog may scoot along on his/her rear because of discomfort. Manual expression of the contents may be accomplished two ways:
  1. Using thumb and index finger, squeeze the two sacs together and up (dorsal).
  2. Insert a lubricated, gloved forefinger into the rectum and locate an anal sac. Apply firm, continuous pressure between the forefinger internally and the thumb on the exterior. Squeezing too hard can damage tissues.

A light tan to dark brown fluid or pasty excretion will squirt from the duct. It may contain particles or, in case of infection, blood and pus.

Circumanal glands extend from the skin into the subcutis superficial to the anal sacs. These strange glands contain sebaceous (oil) glands, but they lack ducts and do not appear to produce a secretion. Their function is unknown. Lumps in the skin in this region in old dogs are caused by benign tumors of the circumanal glands. More rarely, malignant tumors (cancers) may occur in the anal sac walls.

Figure 1

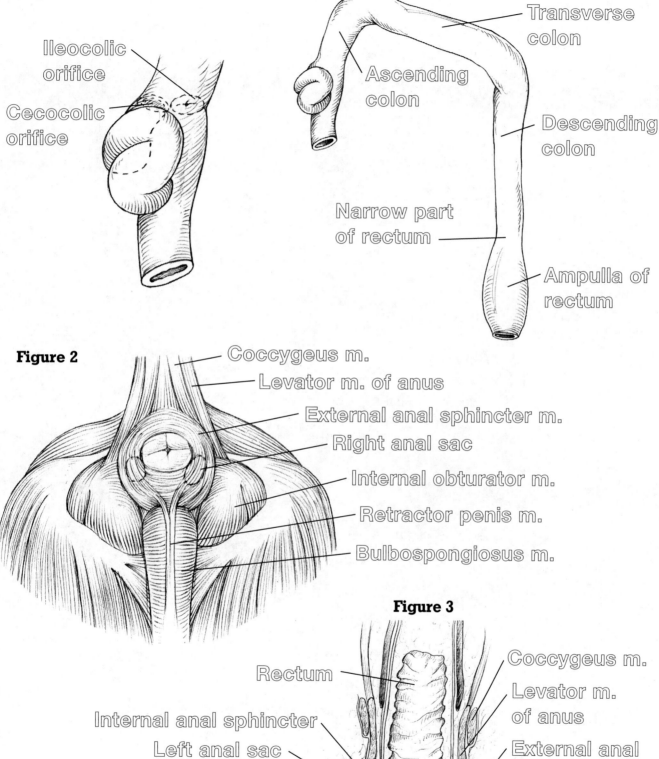

Ileocolic orifice

Cecocolic orifice

Transverse colon

Ascending colon

Descending colon

Narrow part of rectum

Ampulla of rectum

Figure 2

Coccygeus m.

Levator m. of anus

External anal sphincter m.

Right anal sac

Internal obturator m.

Retractor penis m.

Bulbospongiosus m.

Figure 3

Rectum

Internal anal sphincter

Left anal sac

Anal sac duct

Circumanal glands

Anal canal

Coccygeus m.

Levator m. of anus

External anal sphincter m.

Right anal sac

Body Cavities and Serous Membranes

Body Cavities and Serous Membranes

PLATE 56

Diagrammatic drawing of major body cavities lined by serous membranes of the bitch. **Peritoneum** also suspends and encloses some of the male reproductive organs.

Peritoneum is divided into three continuous parts: Color the dashed lines without lifting your pencil from the paper.

1. Parietal peritoneum – lines abdominal cavity and part of pelvic cavity (L, paries = wall).

2. Connecting peritoneum – suspends organs by a double fold that encloses vessels and nerves.
  a. Mes + organ suspended: **mesentery** (G., mesos = middle + enteron = intestine).
  b. Peritoneal ligaments: suspend and support, e.g., **falciform ligament** of liver.

3. Visceral peritoneum - encloses a viscus (L, large internal organ; plural, viscera).

The musculomembranous diaphragm is covered by peritoneum on its abdominal surface; pleura on its thoracic surface.

Pleurae – two serous membranes, each continuous and forming a pleural sac.

1. Parietal pleura – lines each half of thoracic cavity: diaphragmatic pleura, costal pleura and mediastinal pleura

On each side, the mediastinal pleura limits the mediastinum, a space containing the heart, trachea, esophagus, the great blood vessels, nerves, thymus, loose connective tissue and fat.

2. Visceral pleura – covers each lung.

Pericardium

1. Visceral serous pericardium – covers heart muscle and reflects around base of heart and great vessels

2. Parietal serous pericardium – covered by fibrous pericardium that blends with pericardial mediastinal pleura.

Serous cavities: peritoneal cavity, pleural cavity, pericardial cavity.
Fine spaces between parietal and visceral serous membranes containing lubricating serous fluids (resembling blood serum).
Serous fluids increase in inflammatory conditions termed peritonitis, pleuritis and pericarditis.

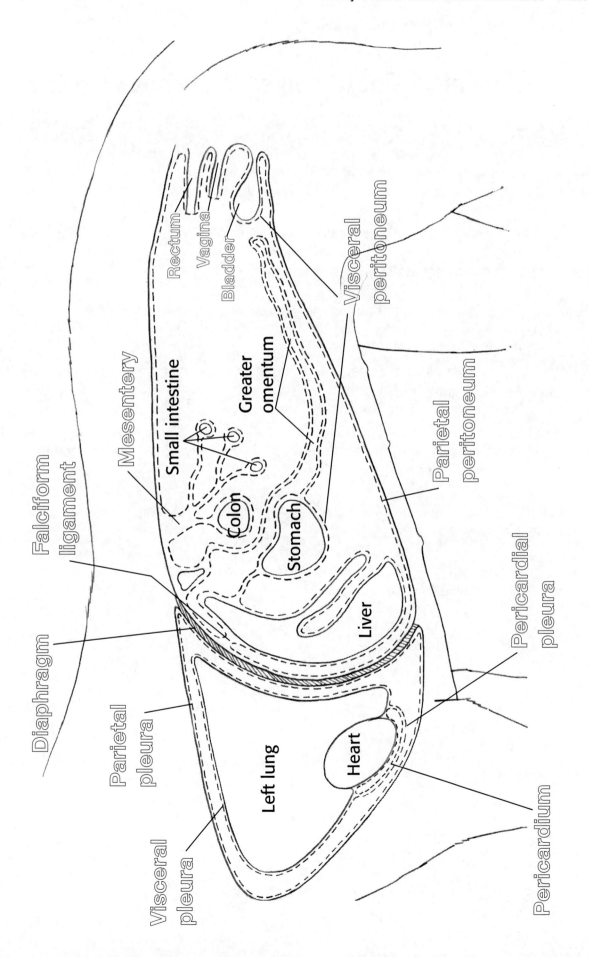

In Place Positions of Internal Organs

PLATE 57

Figure 1. Right lateral view of the internal organs of the bitch.
Figure 2. Left lateral view of the internal organs of the dog.

Color the names and the organs indicated.

The diaphragm is represented by a dashed line.

Relations of organs to each other and to the exterior of the body are important in the following procedures:

1. <u>Palpation</u> – feeling from the exterior or through an organ that opens to the exterior, for example, the rectum.

2. <u>Auscultation</u> – listening to normal and abnormal sounds from internal organs, mainly the lungs, heart, arteries, stomach, and intestines. A <u>stethoscope</u> is a device used to convey these sounds to one's ears.

3. <u>Percussion</u> – striking short, sharp blows on a region and listening for sounds obtained from underlying organs.

4. <u>Surgical</u> <u>approaches</u> to internal organs. A knowledge of these relations is essential for determining where to make incisions.

5. Interpretation of <u>radiographic</u> and <u>ultrasonic</u> <u>images</u>.

Figure 1

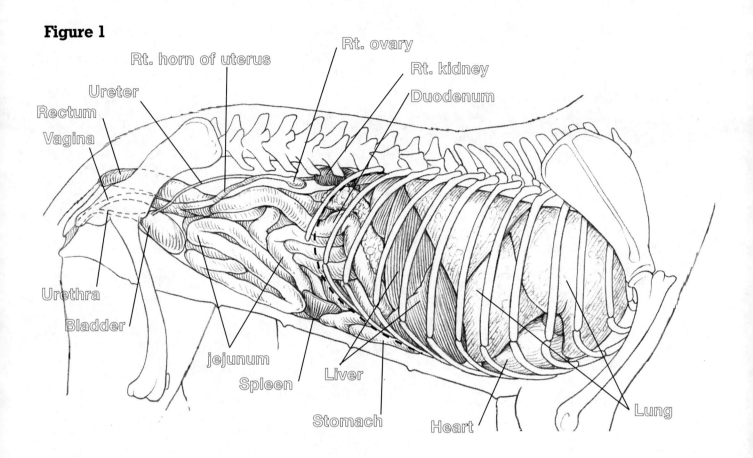

Rt. horn of uterus
Rt. ovary
Rt. kidney
Duodenum
Ureter
Rectum
Vagina
Urethra
Bladder
jejunum
Spleen
Liver
Stomach
Heart
Lung

Figure 2

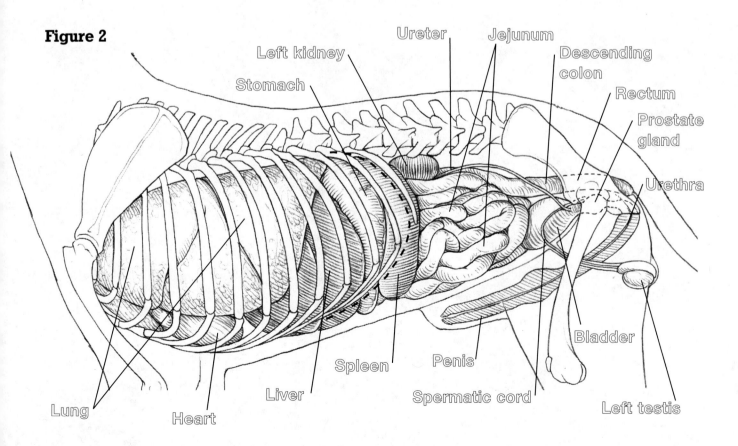

Ureter
Jejunum
Left kidney
Stomach
Descending colon
Rectum
Prostate gland
Urethra
Lung
Heart
Liver
Spleen
Penis
Spermatic cord
Bladder
Left testis

Cardiovascular System

Major Circulatory Patterns

PLATE 58

Color the names of organs and regions.

Coloring the arrows blue, trace the flow of poorly-oxygenated blood:

From the **cranial** and **caudal caval veins** (L., venae cavae) to the **right atrium**

Through the **right atrioventricular valve** to the **right ventricle**

Out of the heart through the **pulmonary trunk valve** into the pulmonary circulation

Through the **pulmonary trunk** and **left and right pulmonary arteries** to the lungs

Finally, to capillaries (smallest blood vessels) in the walls of alveoli (little air sacs) in the lungs. Here carbon dioxide is released from hemoglobin in erythrocytes (red blood cells) and oxygen is bound to the hemoglobin for transport to the body's tissues.

Coloring the arrows red, trace the flow of oxygenated blood:

From capillaries in the lungs, through **pulmonary veins** to the **left atrium**

Through the **left atrioventricular valve** to the **left ventricle**

Then through the **aortic valve** into the **aorta** and the systemic circulation. Color the arrows in arteries red; arrows in veins, blue. Satellite (companion) veins accompany most arteries.

In the hepatic portal system, blood in veins coming from the stomach, pancreas, spleen, and intestines is carried by the **portal vein** to sinusoidal capillaries in the liver. From these capillaries, blood is carried by **hepatic veins** to the **caudal caval vein** (L., vena cava caudalis). Color veins blue.

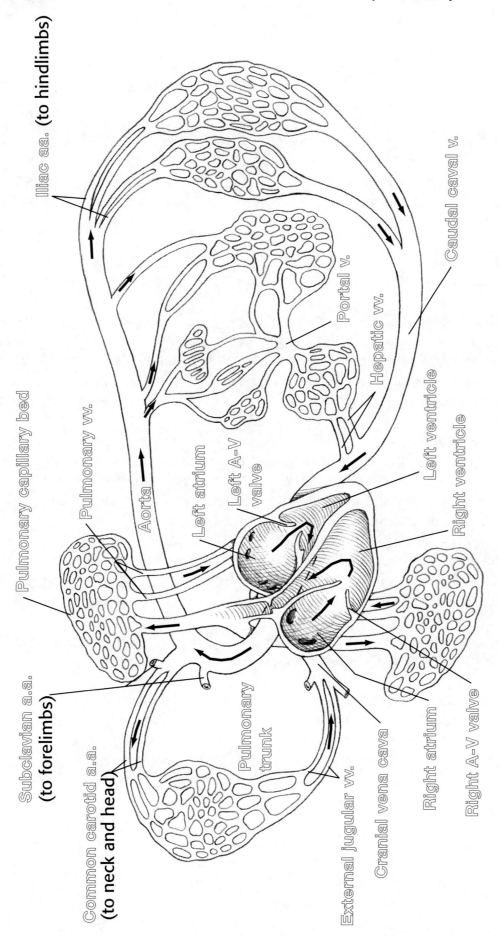

Iliac aa. (to hindlimbs)

Caudal caval v.

Portal v.

Hepatic vv.

Left ventricle

Right ventricle

Pulmonary capillary bed

Pulmonary vv.

Aorta

Left atrium

Left A-V valve

Right A-V valve

Subclavian a.a. (to forelimbs)

Common carotid a.a. (to neck and head)

Pulmonary trunk

External jugular vv.

Cranial vena cava

Right atrium

The Canine Heart

PLATE 59

Figure 1. Left lateral view of isolated heart and great vessels. **Coronary arteries** are the first branches of the aorta. **Auricles** are outpocketings of **atria**. Color the names and structures indicated in these drawings.

Figure 2. Sectioned heart, exposing its chambers. A cardiac skeleton of fibrous tissue and some cartilage separates the cardiac muscle of the atria from that of the ventricles. A-V = atrioventricular

The **arterial ligament** is a remnant of the arterial duct (L., ductus arteriosus) that shunted blood from the pulmonary trunk to the aorta in the fetus (unborn puppy). An oval foramen carried blood from the right atrium to the left atrium in the fetal heart. Most of the blood flowing into the fetal heart is shunted through these two passages, bypassing the pulmonary circulation. Since the fetal lungs are not functioning, mother's blood in the placenta supplies oxygen to the fetus.

The most common congenital vascular defect in dogs is a patent (open) ductus arteriosus (PDA) that persists after birth. It is fairly easy to diagnose, and the condition is correctable. In the latest treatment, a coil is delivered into the duct by an intravenous catheter. A clot formed on the coil will start closure of the duct.

Congenital cardiac defects include valvular insufficiency (incomplete closure), stenosis (constriction of pulmonary or aortic valves), atrial septal defects and ventricular septal defect. Septal defects are abnormal openings in the septa.

During beating of the heart, the two atria fill and contract. Then the two ventricles fill and contract, forcing blood into the pulmonary trunk and the aorta.

Heart sounds are caused by the rush of blood and the closing heart valves, first the A-V valves, then the pulmonary and aortic valves. The sinoatrial node in the wall of the right atrium is the pacemaker (controlled by the nervous system) that begins the rhythmic contractions of the atria. Cardiac muscle fibers conduct impulses to the atrioventricular node in the wall (septum) between the atria. Specialized cardiac muscle fibers (Purkinje fibers) descend from the atrioventricular node to the ventricles, causing their contraction.

Figure 1

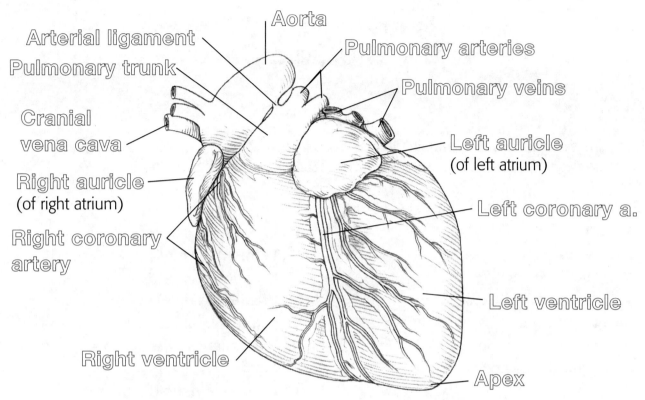

Aorta

Arterial ligament

Pulmonary trunk

Pulmonary arteries

Cranial vena cava

Pulmonary veins

Right auricle (of right atrium)

Left auricle (of left atrium)

Right coronary artery

Left coronary a.

Left ventricle

Right ventricle

Apex

Figure 2

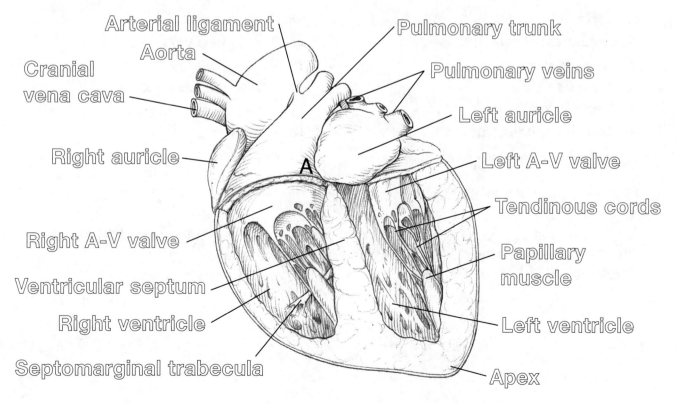

Arterial ligament

Aorta

Pulmonary trunk

Cranial vena cava

Pulmonary veins

Right auricle

Left auricle

Left A-V valve

Tendinous cords

Right A-V valve

Ventricular septum

Papillary muscle

Right ventricle

Left ventricle

Septomarginal trabecula

Apex

A

Vessels and Related Organs
in the Thoracic Cavity

PLATE 60

Underline the **boldfaced names** in different colors and color indicated organs on the drawings. Color arteries red, veins blue, and nerves yellow. Satellite veins not seen here.

Figure 1. Dissected thorax of a dog opened from left side.

1. **Aorta**
2. **L. vagus nerve**
3. **L. subclavian artery**
4. **L. costocervical trunk**
5. **L. vertebral a.**
6. **L. internal thoracic a.**
7. **L. superficial cervical a.**
8. **L. axillary a.**
9. **Brachiocephalic trunk**

10. **L. common carotid a.**
11. **Pulmonary trunk**
12. **L. pulmonary a.**
13. **Cranial caval vein**
14. **L. intercostal aa.**
15. **Pulmonary veins**
16. **Caudal caval vein**
17. **L. phrenic n.** (to diaphragm)
18. **Thoracic duct**

Figure 2. Dissected thorax of a dog opened from right side.

1. **Aorta**
2. **Caudal caval vein**
3. **R. vagus nerve**
4. **Azygous vein**
5. **Cranial caval vein**
6. **Brachiocephalic trunk**
7. **R. vertebral a.**

8. **R. costocervical trunk**
9. **R. common carotid a.**
10. **R. subclavian a.**
11. **R. internal thoracic a.**
12. **R. superficial cervical a.**
13. **R. axillary a.**
14. **R. phrenic n.**

Three passages perforate the **diaphragm**, the musculomembranous partition between the thoracic and abdominal cavities:

Ah. Aortic hiatus – transmits aorta, azygous vein and chyle cistern (beginning of thoracic duct).
Eh. Esophageal hiatus – transmits esophagus and vagus nerves
Fvc. Vena caval foramen (foramen venae cavae) – transmits caudal caval vein.

Figure 1

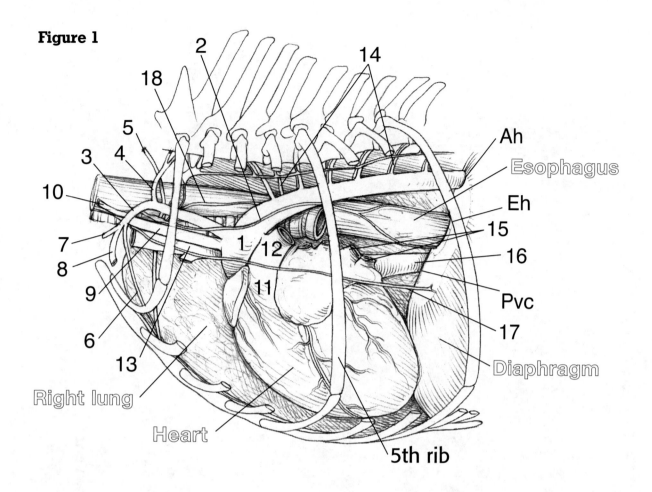

Figure 2

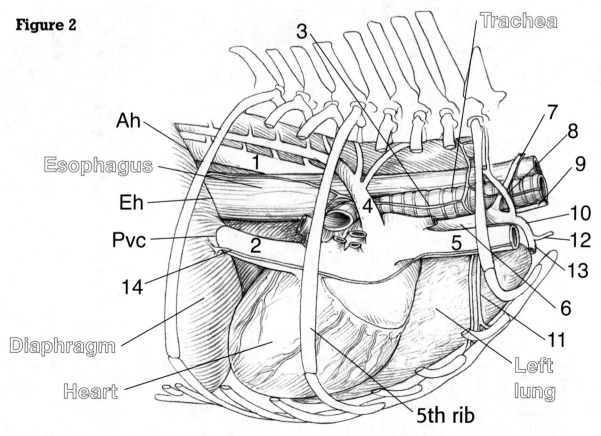

Vessels of the Abdominal Cavity

PLATE 61

Ventral view. Underline the **boldfaced names** of the vessels. Color arteries (a.) red, veins (v.) blue on the drawings.

Figure 1. <u>Branches of aorta</u>:

1. Celiac a.
2. L. gastric a.
3. Esophageal a.
4. Hepatic a.
5. Branches to liver
6. R. gastric a.
7. R. gastroepiploic a.
8. Cranial pancreaticoduodenal a.
9. Splenic a,
10. Branches to pancreas
11. Branches to spleen

12. L. gastroepiploic a.
13. Cranial mesenteric a.
14. Ileocolic a.
15. Middle colic a.
16. R. colic a.
17. Ileal a.
18. Caudal pancreaticoduodenal a.
19. Jejunal aa.
20. L. phrenicoabdominal a.
21. L. renal a.
22. L. ovarian a.(testicular a.)

23. Caudal mesenteric a.
24. Cranial rectal a.
25. L. colic a.

Branches of caudal caval vein:
26. Hepatic vv.
27. L. phrenicoabdominal v.
28. L. renal v.
29. L. ovarian vein (L. testicular v.)
30. R. ovarian v.

Figure 2. <u>Branches of portal vein</u>:

31. Gastroduodenal v.
32. R. gastric v.
33. R. gastroepiploic v.
34. Cranial pancreaticoduodenal v.
35. Splenic v.
36. L. gastric v.

37. L. gastroepiploic v.
38. Branches from spleen
39. Branch from pancreas
40. Ileocolic v.
41. R. colic v.
42. Cranial mesenteric v.

43. Caudal pancreaticoduodenal v.
44. Jejunal vv.
45. Caudal mesenteric v.
46. Middle colic v.
47. L. colic v.

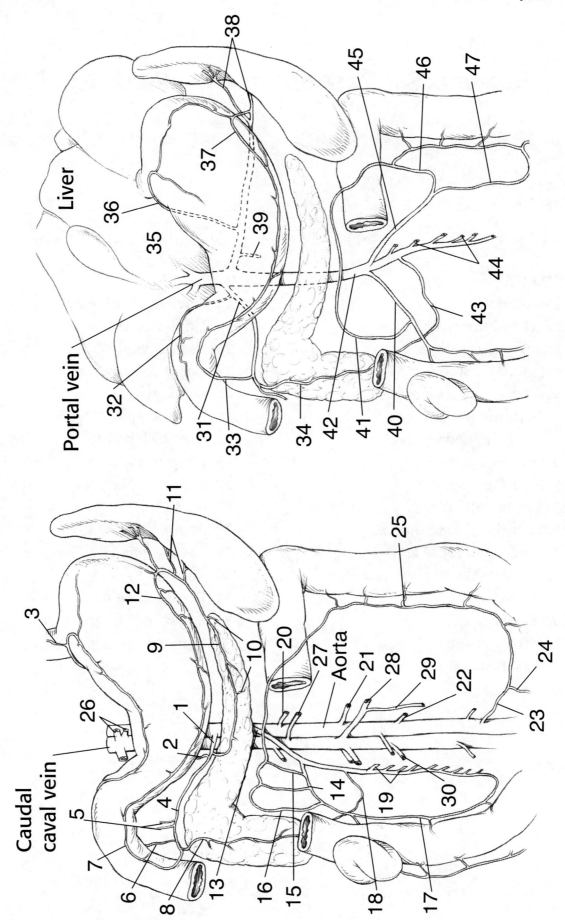

Figure 2

Liver

Portal vein

38

37

36

35

39

45

46

47

44

43

32

31

33

34

42

41

40

Figure 1

Caudal
caval vein

3

26

11

12

9

10

20

27

Aorta

21

28

29

22

25

24

23

1

2

4

5

7

6

8

13

16

15

14

19

30

18

17

Superficial Vessels of the Head and Neck

PLATE 62

Figure 1. Superficial arteries. Right lateral view.
Figure 2. Superficial veins. Right lateral view.

Underline the **boldfaced names** and color each artery (a.) red, each vein(v.) blue.

ARTERIES
1. **Common carotid a.**
2. **Cranial thyroid a.**
3. **Internal carotid a.**
4. **External carotid a.**
5. **Cranial laryngeal a.**
6. **Occipital a.**
7. **Ascending pharyngeal a.**
8. **Lingual a.**
9. **Facial a.**
10. **Caudal auricular a.**
11. **Superficial temporal a..**
12. **Transverse facial a.**
13. **Lat. dorsal palpebral a.**
14. **Lat. ventral palpebral a.**
15. **Maxillary a.**
16. **Infraorbital a.**
17. **Nasal aa.**

VEINS
18. **External jugular v.**
19. **Linguofacial v.**
20. **Lingual vein**
21. **Hyoid venous arch**
22. **Sublingual v.**
23. **Facial v.**
24. **Inferior labial v.**
25. **Deep facial v.**
26. **Superior labial v.**
27. **Nasal vv.**
28. **Angular ocular v.**
29. **Ophthalmic v.**
30. **Maxillary v.**
31. **Great auricular v.**
32. **Superficial temporal v.**
33. **Pterygoid plexus**

Figure 1

Figure 2

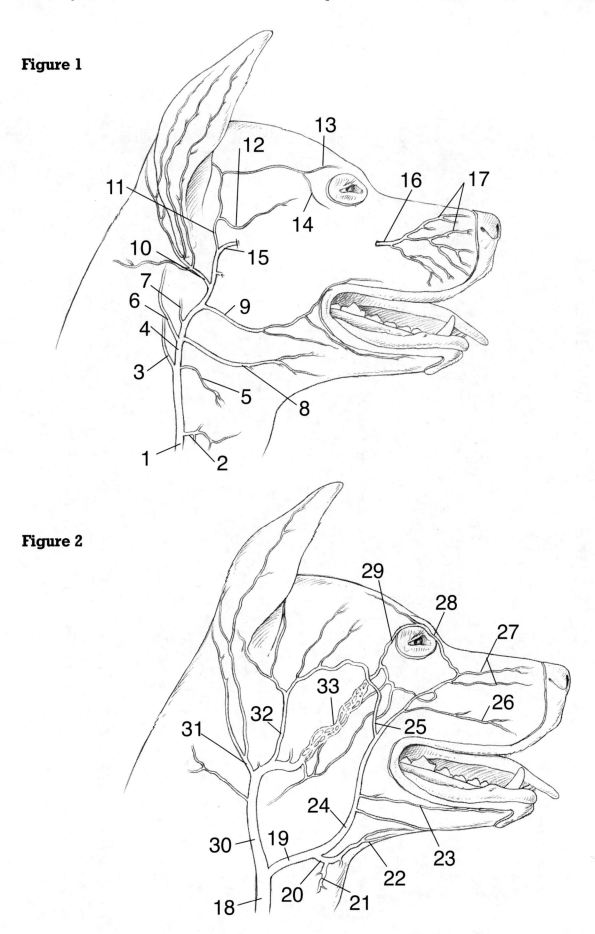

Dog Anatomy - A Coloring Atlas

The Dog's Pulse. Venipuncture Sites

PLATE 63

Figure 1.
A. Taking the dog's pulse by palpating the **femoral artery** just deep to the skin and fascia in the femoral triangle just deep to the skin and fascia on the medial aspect of the upper thigh. The hand is wrapped around the cranial aspect of the thigh.

B. Skin and fascia removed from the medial aspect of the left thigh, exposing the femoral triangle, a space between the caudal belly of the **sartorial m.** cranially and the **pectineal m.** caudally. Fingertips are superimposed over the femoral a.

Figure 2. A large dog lying on the right side with the left elbow moved craniad. The heart beat may be felt (or auscultated) in the fifth and sixth intercostal spaces just dorsal to the sternum.

Figure 3. Site for venipuncture of the cranial branch of the lateral **saphenous vein.**

Figure 4. Site for venipuncture of the **cephalic vein.**

Color the names and the structures indicated, coloring the femoral artery and the heart red, veins blue, and muscles pink.

The pulse is the rhythmic expansion of an artery that may be felt with the fingers. The pulse rate reflects the heart rate – the number of heart beats per minute. The normal resting heart rate of dogs varies between 75 and 120 beats per minute. The heart beat may be felt in smaller dogs by grasping around the sternum with the thumb on one side and fingers on the opposite side.

Tachycardia is the term for an excessively rapid heart beat. Bradycardia is an abnormal slowing of the heart beat. An abnormal sound coming from the heart is termed a murmur. It may be an "innocent murmur", or it may indicate an abnormal condition of the heart.

The veins at the venipuncture sites lie immediately deep to the skin, subcutis, and fascia. Small branches of the medial cutaneous antebrachial nerve parallel the cephalic vein. Sensation to the lateral skin of the leg is provided by branches from the superficial peroneal and lateral cutaneous sural nerves.

Compression of a vein proximal to the site of venipuncture, distends the vein and makes it easier to insert a needle or catheter (long plastic tube). Compression is released for injection. The femoral vein may be used for venipuncture without compression proximal to the needle.

Cardiovascular System

The Dog's Pulse. Venipuncture Sites - **Plate 63**

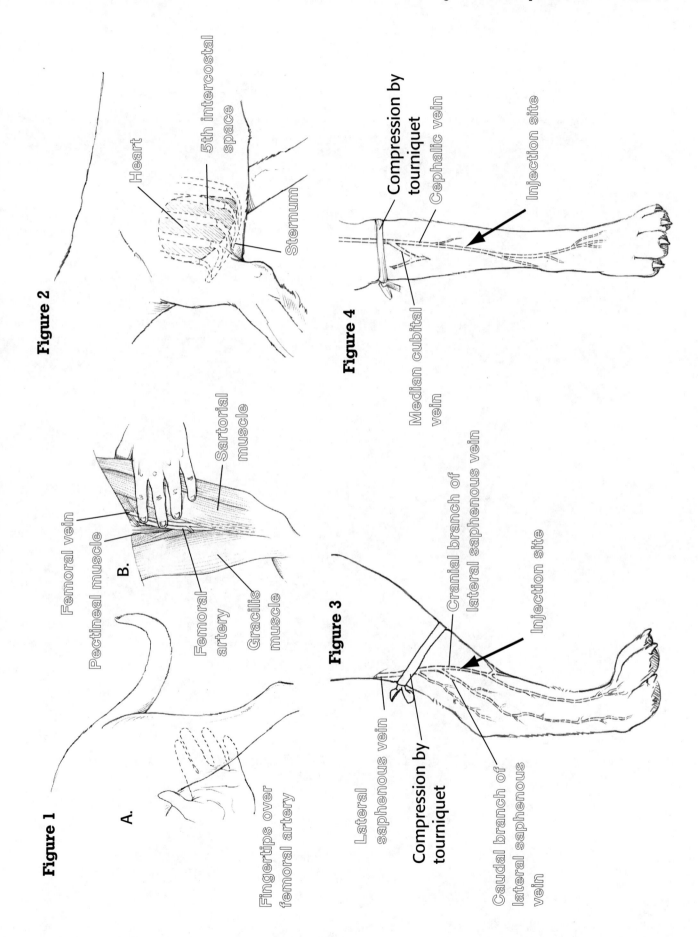

Figure 1

A.

Fingertips over femoral artery

Femoral vein

Pectineal muscle

B.

Femoral artery

Gracilis muscle

Sartorial muscle

Figure 2

Heart

5th intercostal space

Sternum

Figure 3

Lateral saphenous vein

Compression by tourniquet

Caudal branch of lateral saphenous vein

Cranial branch of lateral saphenous vein

Injection site

Figure 4

Compression by tourniquet

Cephalic vein

Injection site

Median cubital vein

Immune System

Bone Marrow, Thymus, and Spleen

PLATE 64

Organs of the immune system produce cells and their products that combat bacteria, viruses, and cancer cells.

Color the names and the drawings of these organs indicated on the drawing.

Red bone marrow produces red blood cells (erythrocytes), white blood cells (leukocytes – neutrophils, eosinophils, basophils, lymphocytes, monocytes, and platelets). Platelets are fragments of large cells (megakarocytes) in bone marrow that are essential for blood clotting. Red marrow occupies spaces in spongy bone in long bones, vertebrae, ribs, sternebrae, and flat bones. Sternebrae and the wing of the ilium are sites for obtaining bone marow samples.

Yellow bone marrow in the medullary cavity consists primarily of fat cells, but blood-cell-producing units of stem cells can begin to generate blood cells again in some cases of anemia (lack of quality or quantity of red blood cells). Production of abnormal leukocytes is termed leukemia.

The **thymus** continues to grow until puberty, occupying the cranial part of the mediastinum and extending through the thoracic inlet into the neck next to the trachea. Then it gradually becomes smaller (involutes), persisting as a small organ in the cranial part of the mediastinum in the adult. The thymus produces white blood cells called T-cell lymphocytes. These cells populate the spleen and lymph nodes.

Since it is attached to the stomach by the greater omentum, the position of the **spleen** in the left side of the abdominal cavity changes slightly as the stomach changes shape or the spleen swells with blood. At first blush, the reddish-brown color of the spleen exposed to air is because of the blood-engorged red pulp. The capsule and trabeculae (little beams) of the canine spleen contain smooth muscle that contracts to move stored blood into the circulation. Other functions of the spleen include: 1. Formation of red blood cells in the fetus; 2. Destruction of old red blood cells and particles in the blood; 3. Production of lymphocytes in the white pulp; 4. Production of platelets by megakaryocytes.

The spleen is not essential to life, and it may be removed surgically if it grows abnormally large or if it ruptures.

Spleen

Rib 13

Thymus (in puppy)

Thymus (in adult)

Yellow bone marrow

Red bone marrow

Lymph Nodes and Lymph Vessels

PLATE 65

A **lymphocenter (lc.)** is a **lymph node (ln.)** or a group of lymph nodes that receive lymphatic (lymph) vessels draining a given region of the body. A fraction of tissue fluid that is not returned to blood capillaries is moved by tissue pressure forces into lymph capillaries and then into larger lymphatics. Lymph within these vessels filters through a series of lymph nodes and connecting lymph vessels that eventually return lymph to the large veins. Phagocytes (cell-eating cells) in lymph nodes remove foreign particles, bacteria, and cancer cells from lymph. Lymph nodes also produce lymphocytes.

Underline the names and color the lymphocenters (lc) and lymph vessels on the drawing. Arrows indicate lymph flow.

1. **Parotid lc.** – one ln.
2. **Mandibular lc.** – 2 –3 lnn.
3. **Retropharyngeal lc.** – medial ln. larger
4. **Deep cervical lc.** Cranial, middle and caudal cervical lnn.
5. **Left tracheal trunk**
6. **Superficial cervical lc.**
7. **Right lymphatic trunk**
8. **Dorsal thoracic lc.**
9. **Thoracic duct** – Empties into cranial caval vein
10. **Bronchial lc.** – Tracheobronchial lnn., pulmonary lnn.
11. **Mediastinal lc.** – Cranial, middle, and caudal mediastinal lnn.
12. **Ventral thoracic lc.** – Sternal lnn.
13. **Axillary lc.** – Axillary and accessory axillary lnn.

14. **Chyle cistern** – Receives lymphatic trunks Origin of thoracic duct
15. **Celiac lc.** – Hepatic lnn., gastric lnn., splenic lnn., pancreaticoduodenal lnn.
16. **Cranial mesenteric lc.** – Jejunal lnn., Right, middle and left colic lnn.
17. **Lumbar lc.** – Lumbar aortic lnn., renal lnn.
18. **Lumbar trunks**
19. **Intestinal trunks**
20. **Iliosacral lc.** – Medial iliac lnn., sacral lnn., hypogastric lnn.,
21. **Iliofemoral lc.** – Illiofemoral ln. Femoral ln., – small and inconstant
22. **Superficial inguinal lc.** – Scrotal lnn. in male. Mammary lnn. in female
23. **Popliteal lc.** – one large ln.

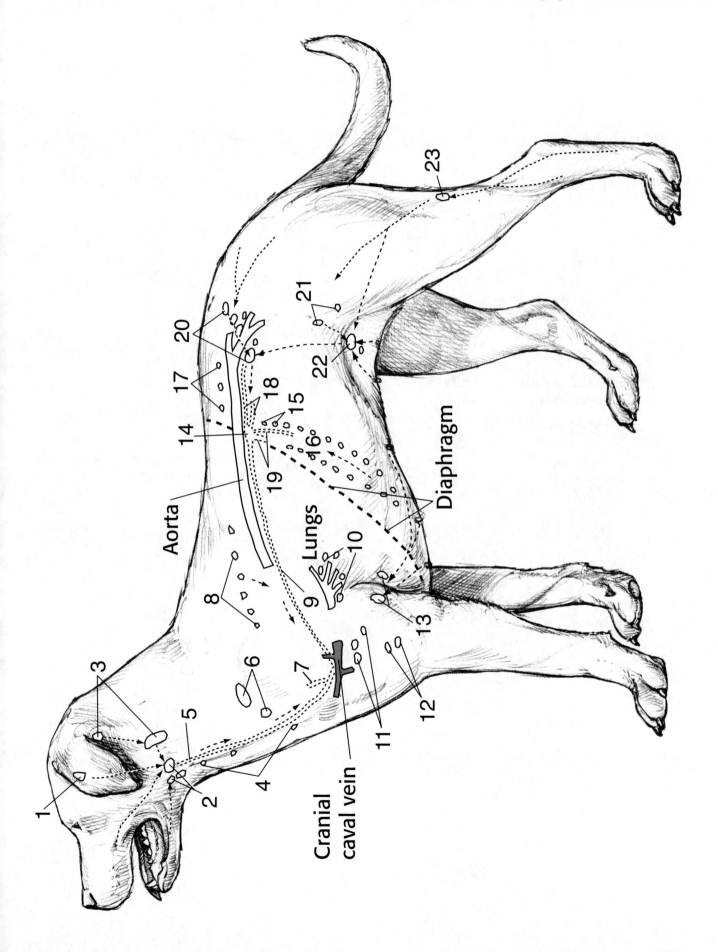

Aorta

Diaphragm

Lungs

Cranial
caval vein

1
2
3
4
5
6
7
8
9
10
11
12
13
14
15
16
17
18
19
20
21
22
23

Tonsils

PLATE 66

In this drawing, the root of the tongue is depressed to visualize the **palatine tonsils**, each slightly protruding from a <u>tonsillar</u> <u>sinus</u>.

Color the names and the structures indicated.

A tonsil is a small mass of lymphoid tissue under the mucous membrane. Efferent lymphatic vessels carry lymph and lymphocytes from tonsils.

The dog has three pairs of tonsils:
1. **Palatine tonsils** – in the lateral walls of the oropharynx .
2. <u>Pharyngeal</u> <u>tonsils</u> (<u>adenoids</u>) – lymphatic nodules in the nasopharynx. (Not seen here.)
3. <u>Lingual</u> <u>tonsils</u> – diffuse in the base of the tongue. Not visible grossly.

When the palatine tonsils are inflamed (<u>tonsillitis</u>), greatly enlarged and painful, the dog has difficulty swallowing and will refuse to eat.

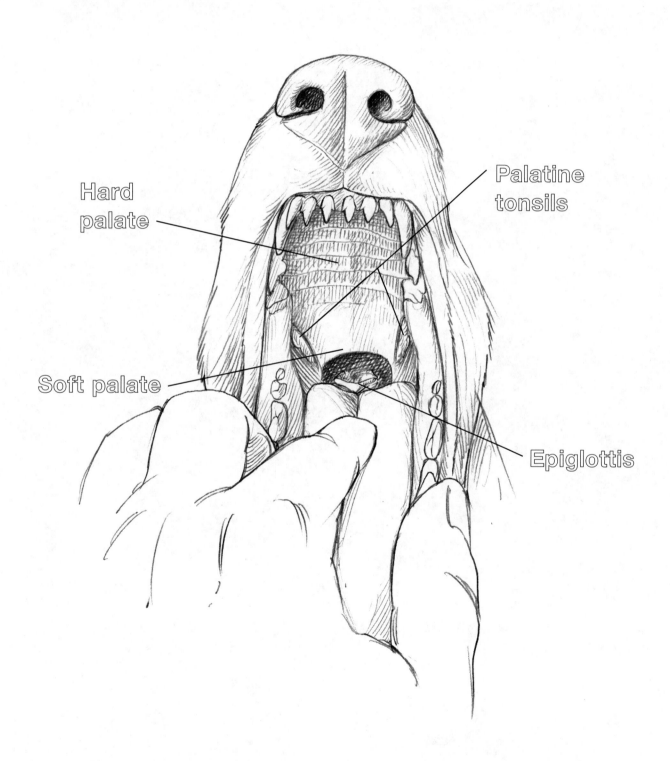

Hard palate

Palatine tonsils

Soft palate

Epiglottis

Respiratory System

Nasal Cavity and Nasopharynx

PLATE 67

Figure 1. Sagittal section of the dog's head with the nasal septum removed, revealing the interior of the left nasal fossa (half of the nasal cavity).

Color the names on the drawings and the structures indicated.

A short arrow indicates the entrance to the <u>auditory</u> <u>tube</u> that connects with the tympanic cavity of the middle ear, admitting air into the middle ear. This anatomic arrangement serves to equalize air pressure on each side of the eardrum.

Trace the long arrow indicating the flow of inspired air.

For a view of the nasal septum, see Plate 43.

There are three pharynges (plural of pharynx): **1. Oropharynx** ventral to the soft palate, **2. nasopharynx** dorsal to the soft palate, extending caudad from the choanae (exits from the nasal fossa on each side), **3. laryngopharynx** dorsal to the larynx and leading into the esophagus.

In this drawing, the soft palate is in the breathing position, directing air into the larynx. For a description of the changes in positions of the tongue, soft palate, and epiglottis during swallowing, see Plate 51.

An abnormality, <u>dorsal</u> <u>displacement</u> <u>of</u> <u>the</u> <u>soft</u> <u>palate</u>, prevents the soft palate from returning to the normal breathing position after swallowing has occurred. Surgical correction is indicated.

Figure 2. Dissection showing the **lateral nasal gland** in the **maxillary recess** (the maxillary sinus of the dog) in the maxilla, the course of the duct of this gland, and the course of the **nasolacrimal duct** carrying tears from the conjunctival sac in front of the eye. The function of the watery secretion of the lateral nasal gland is to help cool the body when the dog pants. The copious secretion when the dog is hot cools the inspired air. It also humidifes the air. Color the names and structures indicated. Trace the courses of the ducts.

Figure 1

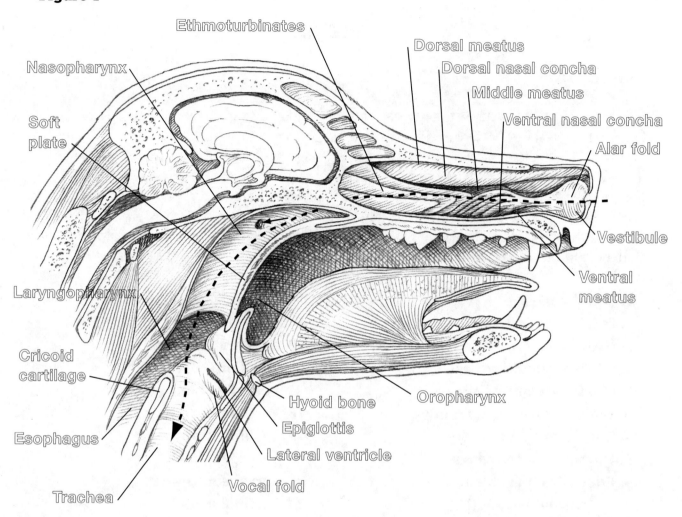

Ethmoturbinates

Dorsal meatus

Dorsal nasal concha

Middle meatus

Ventral nasal concha

Alar fold

Nasopharynx

Soft plate

Vestibule

Laryngopharynx

Ventral meatus

Cricoid cartilage

Oropharynx

Hyoid bone

Epiglottis

Esophagus

Lateral ventricle

Trachea

Vocal fold

Figure 2

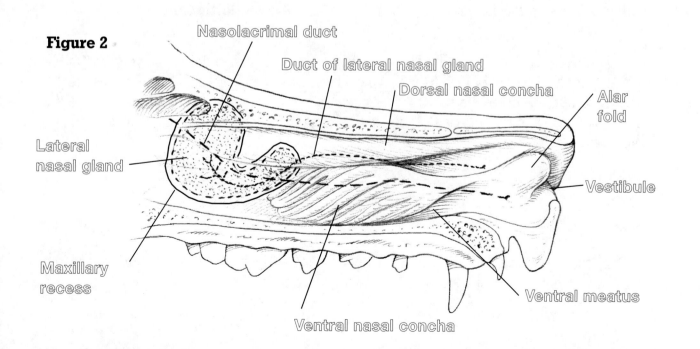

Nasolacrimal duct

Duct of lateral nasal gland

Dorsal nasal concha

Alar fold

Lateral nasal gland

Vestibule

Maxillary recess

Ventral meatus

Ventral nasal concha

Larynx

PLATE 68

Figure 1. Right lateral view of laryngeal cartilages and cranial tracheal rings.
Figure 2. Dorsal view of larynx. Pharynx and esophagus cut mid-dorsally.
Figure 3. Right lateral view of laryngeal muscles. Right half of thyroid cartilage; thyroarytenoid muscle and most of cricothyroid muscle removed.
Figure 4. Median section of the larynx. A dashed line indicates extent of the laryngeal ventricle.

Three regions of the laryngeal cavity are: **A. vestibule, B. glottis, and C. infraglottic cavity**
Underline the **boldfaced names** and color indicated structures on the drawings.

1. **Hyoid bones**
2. **Epiglottic cartilage**
3. **Hyoepglottic m.**
4. **Interarytenoid cartilage**
5. **Right arytenoid cartilage**
6. **Thyroid cartilage, 6a = edge**
7. **Cricoid cartilage**
8. **Trachea, tracheal rings**
9. **Cricothyroid ligament**
10. **Thyrohyoid ligament**
11. **Processes of arytenoid cartilage**
12. **Transverse arytenoid m.**

13. **Dorsal cricoarytenoid m.**
14. **Lateral cricoarytenoid m.**
15. **Cricoarytenoid m.** (stump)
16. **Vocal m.**
17. **Vocal ligament**
18. **Vestibular ligament**
19. **Vestibular m.**
20. **Laryngeal inlet**
21. **Laryngeal ventricle**
22. **Vestibular fold**
23. **Vocal fold**
24. **Aryepiglottic fold**

On each side, a cranial laryngeal nerve (from the vagus n.) supplies the cricothyroid m. and sends an internal sensory branch to the laryngeal mucous membrane. The caudal laryngeal nerve is the termination of the recurrent laryngeal n. that ascends from the vagus n. in the the thorax. All of the intrinsic muscles of the larynx except the cricothyroid muscles receive their motor supply from the caudal laryngeal nerves.

Functions of the larynx:
1. Regulates the volume of air passing through in inspiration and expiration.
2. Prevents foreign material from entering the trachea through partial closure by the epiglottis and constriction of the glottis.
3. Phonation (vocalization) – barking, baying, growling and whining caused by variations in air flow, vibrations of vocal folds and air in laryngeal ventricles.

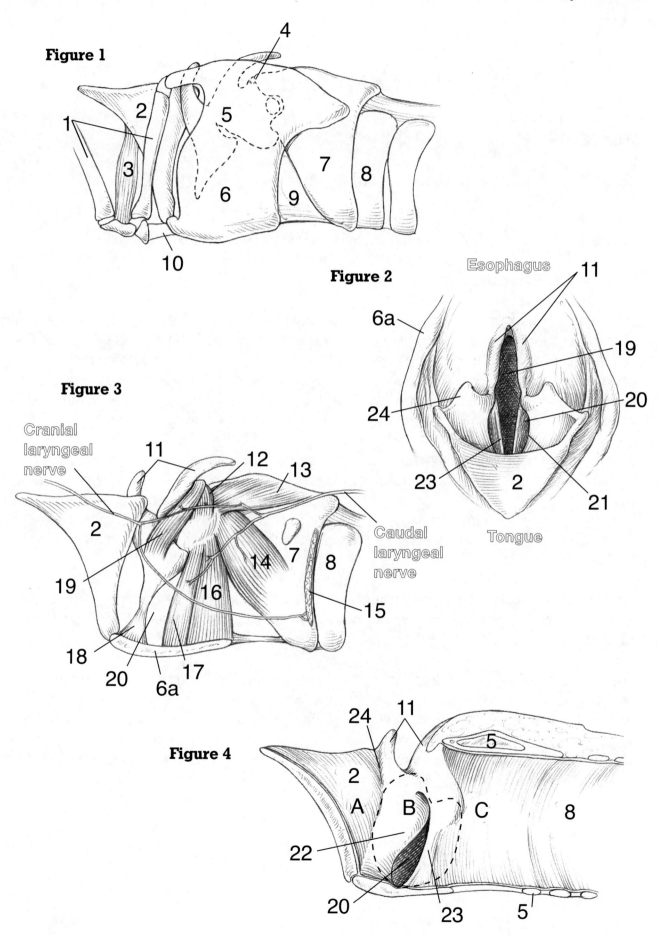

Figure 1

4

2

1

5

3

7

8

6

9

10

Figure 2

Esophagus

6a

11

19

24

20

23

2

21

Tongue

Figure 3

Cranial
laryngeal
nerve

11

12

13

2

Caudal
laryngeal
nerve

19

7

14

8

15

16

18

20   6a   17

Figure 4

24   11

2   5

A   B   C   8

22

20   23   5

Trachea and Lungs

PLATE 69

Figure 1. Dorsal view of **trachea** and **lungs**. Lobes of lungs separated. Diagrammatic drawing of **bronchial tree**.
Figure 2. Cross section of a **tracheal ring**.
Figure 3. Microscopic view of **alveoli** (L., little hollows), tiny air sacs with capillaries in their walls.

Color the names and the structures indicated on the drawings.

The trachea extends from the cricoid cartilage through the neck into the mediastinum to the bifurcation (fork) dorsal to the base of the heart. It consists of around 34 incomplete C-shaped rings of cartilage. Dorsally, the open part of each ring is closed by smooth muscle, the **tracheal muscle**, and fibrous connective tissue. Longitudinal ligaments of fibroelastic connective tissue connect the rings. This tissue continues under the mucous membrane of the two **principal bronchi**, gradually becoming thinner in the smaller conducting airways.

Where the trachea bifurcates into left and right principal bronchi, gaps in the free ends of the tracheal rings are filled by plates of cartilage. Cartilaginous plates continue on to support the walls of the bronchi (singular – bronchus) They are not present in the smallest airways, the bronchioles. Smooth muscle in the walls of airways serve to constrict them. Glands and cells in the mucous membrane produce mucus. Beginning with the nasal cavity, cilia on the cells lining the airways move mucus toward the exterior.

A **terminal bronchiole** leads to respiratory bronchioles. Gas exchange of carbon dioxide from red blood cells and oxygen into them takes place between air within **alveoli** and blood within capillaries in alveolar walls.

The normal breathing rate of dogs varies with their size; smaller dogs breathing more rapidly. The rate may be affected by excitement, exercise, age, illness, environmental temperature, pregnancy, and a full digestive tract. Rapid breathing or panting serves to cool the body by increased dead-space ventilation -- the volume of air that does not take part in gas exchange over a given period. The increased movement of air evaporates mucus in the oral cavity, helping to cool the body. This compensates for the lack of liquid sweat on canine skin.

Figure 1

Figure 2

Figure 3

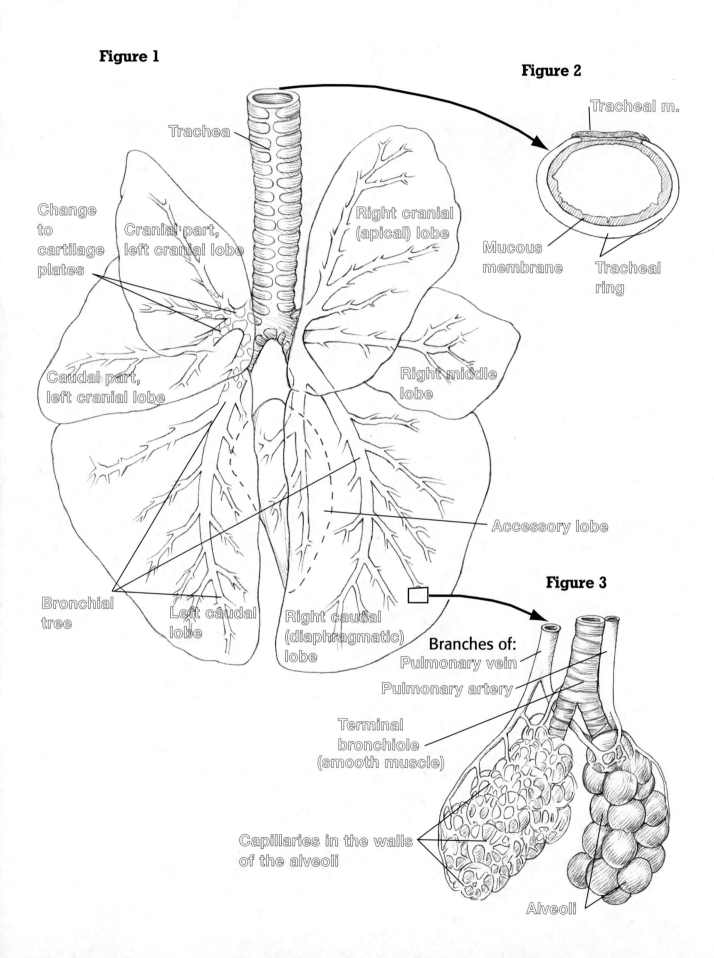

Trachea

Change to cartilage plates

Cranial part, left cranial lobe

Right cranial (apical) lobe

Caudal part, left cranial lobe

Right middle lobe

Bronchial tree

Left caudal lobe

Right caudal (diaphragmatic) lobe

Accessory lobe

Tracheal m.

Mucous membrane

Tracheal ring

Branches of:

Pulmonary vein

Pulmonary artery

Terminal bronchiole (smooth muscle)

Capillaries in the walls of the alveoli

Alveoli

Urinary System

Kidneys, Ureters, Bladder, and Urethra

PLATE 70

Figure 1. Ventral view of urinary organs and associated organs of the female. For differences in the male dog, see Plate 77.
Figure 2. Frontal section of right kidney.

Color the names and the structures indicated on the plate in the same colors.

Millions of microscopic tubular structures called <u>nephrons</u> are located in the **cortex** and **medulla** of the **kidney**. The urine-producing nephrons are closely associated with the extensive blood supply to the kidney. <u>Collecting</u> <u>ducts</u> extend from nephrons to the renal crest, emptying urine into the **pelvis** of the kidney. The pelvis is essentially the beginning of the **ureter**.

Urine is a solution of the products of nitrogen and sulfur <u>metabolism</u> (the processing of substances, mainly nutrients, by the various tissues of the body), Urine also contains inorganic salts, pigments, and the products of toxins inactivated by the liver and excreted by the kidneys. Kidneys regulate the normal levels of substances in the blood such as water, inorganic salts and glucose (blood sugar). In diabetes, the kidneys cannot return excess levels of glucose to the blood, and it spills over into the urine.

Like the nearby **adrenal glands**, kidneys are also endocrine organs. One product regulates blood pressure; another initiates red blood cell production.

Canine urine is watery and yellow. When more water is consumed, urine is diluted and paler. The volume of water excreted varies with water and food consumption, physical activity and environmental temperature. The volume of urine excreted each day is from .03 to 1.6 ounces per pound of body weight.

<u>Urinary</u> <u>calculi</u> (L., pebbles), commonly called kidney and bladder stones or gravel, are abnormal concretions of inorganic salts. They often occur in dogs.

The urinary bladder has two functions:
1. It is a reservoir that expands to contain the urine that is continuously passed to it through the ureters from the kidneys.
2. When a male dog marks his territory, when some dogs are frightened, or a puppy is excited, the bladder voids urine. Smooth muscle fibers of the <u>detrusor</u> <u>muscle</u> in the bladder wall contract and the striated muscle in the wall of the urethra relaxes. Neural control of the bladder is complex.

Figure 1

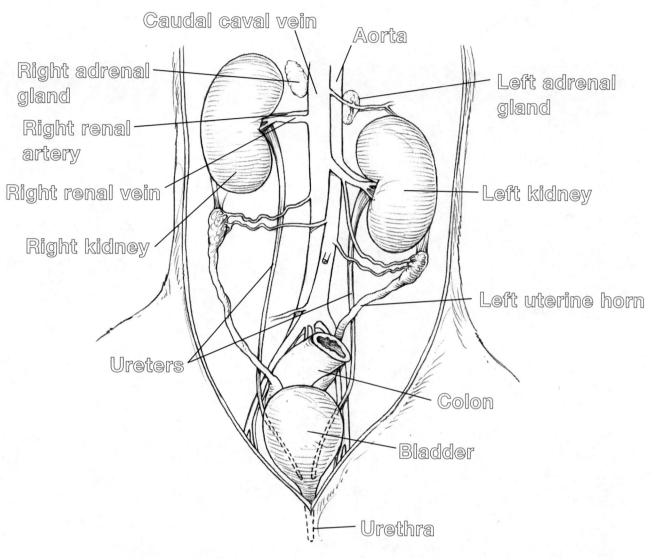

Caudal caval vein

Aorta

Right adrenal gland

Left adrenal gland

Right renal artery

Right renal vein

Left kidney

Right kidney

Left uterine horn

Ureters

Colon

Bladder

Urethra

Figure 2

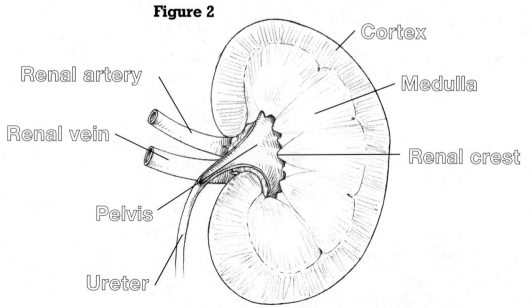

Cortex

Renal artery

Medulla

Renal vein

Renal crest

Pelvis

Ureter

Female Reproductive System

Vulva and Vagina

PLATE 71

Figure 1. Caudal view of **perineum** between **anus** and **vulva**. The vulva consists of two **labia** (L., lips) and the **clitoris**. The clitoris is homologous with the penis of the male, and rarely contains a small clitoral bone.

Figure 2. Dorsal view of opened vulva and **vagina** (L., sheath). The **external uterine opening** of the **cervix** can not be seen, since it faces ventral. The **bladder** is displaced to one side.

Figure 3. Lateral view of vagina, vulva, and related organs. Notice the following:
- Ventral projection of the cervix into the **fornix** of the vagina.
- **Dorsal median postcervical fold**. A speculum (viewing tube) inserted into the vagina may distort this fold into a misleading appearance resembling the vaginal portion of the cervix, with a ventral fissure looking like the external uterine opening.
- Ventral slope of the caudal vagina and the **vaginal vestibule**.

Using different colors, color the names and the structures indicated.

When a bitch (female dog) is in <u>heat</u> (estrus, male dogs attracted), the labia are swollen and a variable amount of blood-tinged mucus is discharged. The odor of a bitch in heat is sensed from quite a distance by the dog's vomeronasal organs (see Plate 43). During estrus (latter part of heat), when oocytes are discharged from the ovary, the bitch will accept mating. The change from proestrus to estrus is best determined by examining the cell types in a smear from the vagina. In the reproductive cycle, the bitch is in proestrus and estrus roughly three times every two years. The interval between heat periods may vary in a given individual.

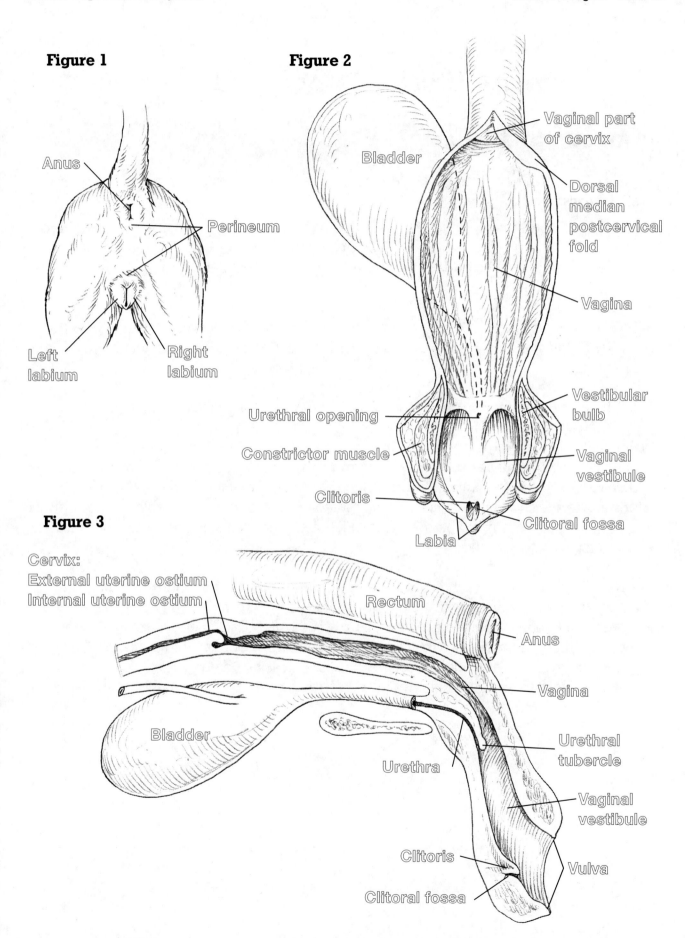

Figure 1

Anus

Perineum

Left labium

Right labium

Figure 2

Bladder

Vaginal part of cervix

Dorsal median postcervical fold

Vagina

Urethral opening

Vestibular bulb

Constrictor muscle

Vaginal vestibule

Clitoris

Clitoral fossa

Labia

Figure 3

Cervix:
External uterine ostium
Internal uterine ostium

Rectum

Anus

Vagina

Bladder

Urethral tubercle

Urethra

Vaginal vestibule

Clitoris

Vulva

Clitoral fossa

Uterus, Uterine Tubes, and Ovaries

PLATE 72

Figure 1. Ventral view of uterus, uterine tubes, ovarian bursae (containing ovaries), and related organs.

The uterus consists of right and left **horns** (L., cornua uteri), **body** (L., corpus uteri), and **neck** (L., cervix uteri). Notice the followinng: The **left ovarian vein** joins the left renal vein, while the right ovarian vein joins the **caudal caval vein**; the ovarian and uterine vessels anastomose (join together).

Figure 2. Ovary exposed by cutting and pulling away the ovarian bursa and uterine tube (oviduct or salpinx). The ovarian bursa is part of the mesosalpinx (the peritoneal fold that suspends the uterine tube).

Color the names and the structures indicated in the figures, using different colors.

When a bitch is spayed (ovariohysterectomized), an incision is made through the ventral abdominal wall. The **suspensory ligaments of the ovaries** are cut, and the **ovarian arteries** and **veins** are ligated (tied off). The **broad ligament** (mesometrium) is incised longitudinally. **Uterine arteries** and **veins** are ligated along with the body of the uterus which is then crushed and cut cranial to the cervix. The ovaries, uterine tubes, and uterus are removed, and the body wall is sutured (sewn) closed.

In Figure 2, notice how close the **ovary** is to the **opening of the uterine tube**. During estrus (in the latter part of heat), oocytes (egg cells) produced by rupture of ovarian follicles are moved into the uterine tube by **fimbriae**, enclosing folds lined with ciliated cells. If spermatozoa (or sperm cells) from the male have made their way to the beginning part of the uterine tube, fertilization (a sperm cell uniting with an oocyte) occurs. A resultant embryo is a ball of dividing cells, a morula. It takes about a week for morulae to pass through the uterine tubes to the cavities of uterine horns.

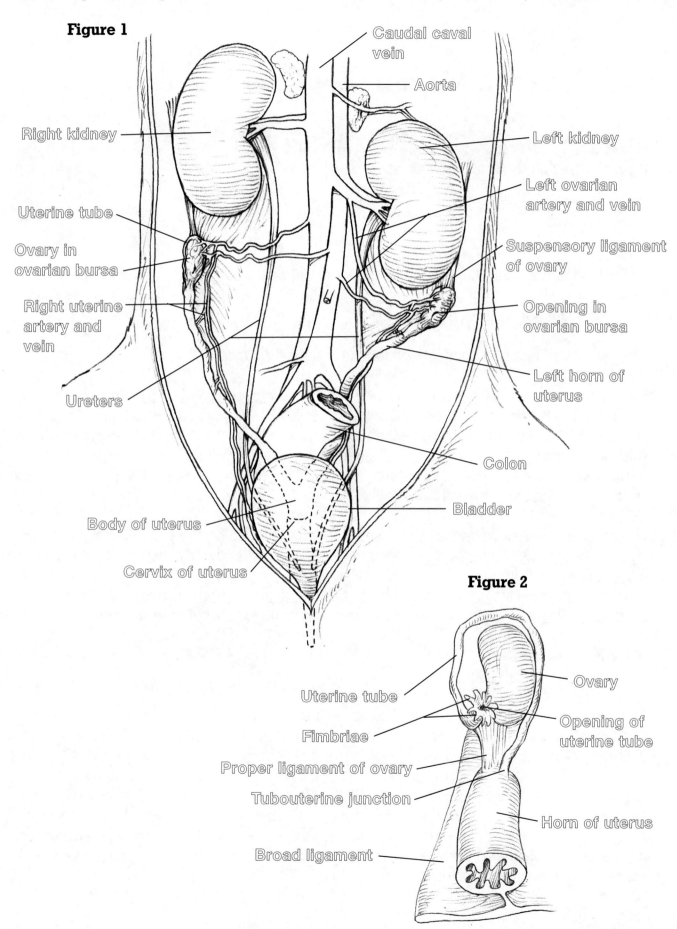

Figure 1

Caudal caval vein

Aorta

Right kidney

Left kidney

Left ovarian artery and vein

Uterine tube

Ovary in ovarian bursa

Suspensory ligament of ovary

Right uterine artery and vein

Opening in ovarian bursa

Left horn of uterus

Ureters

Colon

Bladder

Body of uterus

Cervix of uterus

Figure 2

Uterine tube

Ovary

Fimbriae

Opening of uterine tube

Proper ligament of ovary

Tubouterine junction

Horn of uterus

Broad ligament

Fetal Membranes. The Placenta

PLATE 73

Figure 1. Sectioned blastula (blastocyst).

Upon arriving in the uterus, each morula develops into a blastula that continues to develop as it floats free in the uterus for another week. The embryos become distributed evenly between the two uterine horns.

In the blastula stage, the **inner cell mass** of stem cells is the early embryo. Cells of the **trophoblast** will form the chorionic epithelium of the chorioallantois. The **zona pellucida**, which surrounded the oocyte, soon disintegrates.

Color names and structures indicated here and in the following figures.

Figure 2. Lateral view of a later embryo and developing extraembryonic membranes. At first and continuing on, the embryo is nourished by blood vessels of the **yolk sac**, the first membrane to grow out from the primitive gut. A remnant of the yolk sac persists until birth. **Chorioamniotic folds** meet and break through, forming the **chorion** and the **amnion** that encloses the amniotic cavity around the **embryo**. The **allantois** grows out (arrows) from the primitive gut and joins the **chorion**, forming the **chorioallantois**. Fluid accumulates in the cavities.

Figure 3. Extraembryonic membranes, zonary placenta, and fetus. The process of implantation starts at the end of the free period and lasts a few days. Part of the chorioallantois adheres to the endometrium (uterine lining) in a zonary fashion. Chorionic epithelial cells (trophoblast cells) destroy endometrial tissues to come in contact with maternal capillaries. Fetal blood is in the allantoic capillaries of the chorioallantois. This region is the intricate **placental zone**.

Marginal hematomas along each side are masses of maternal blood. Thus, a placenta consists of two parts: fetal and maternal.

Transfer of nutrients and oxygen from the mother's blood passes through maternal capillaries and trophoblast cells to fetal capillaries; waste materials and carbon dioxide pass in the opposite direction. Normally, fetal blood and maternal blood never mix.

Figure 4. Canine zonary placenta at term. Obtained by surgical delivery (Cesarean section or C-section). Marginal hematomas now appear green because of the decomposition of blood pigment. Color names and the structures indicated, using green for the **marginal hematomas** and red for the **placental zone**. This green pigment is often seen on the fur around the vulva following delivery of the puppies.

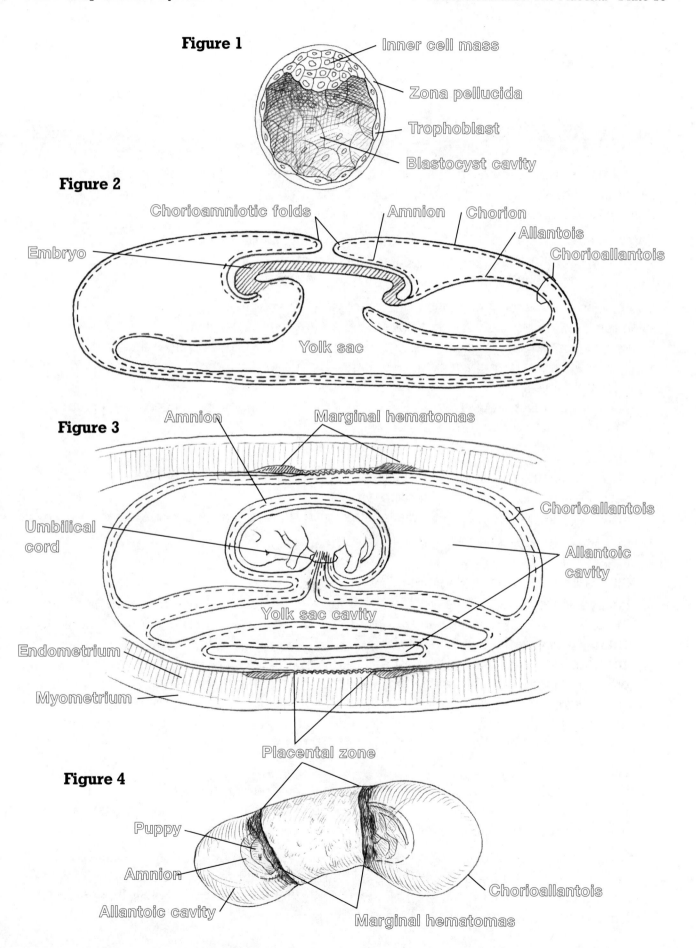

Figure 1

Inner cell mass
Zona pellucida
Trophoblast
Blastocyst cavity

Figure 2

Chorioamniotic folds   Amnion   Chorion
                                               Allantois
                                               Chorioallantois
Embryo
Yolk sac

Figure 3

Amnion   Marginal hematomas
                                    Chorioallantois
Umbilical
cord
                                    Allantoic
                                    cavity
Yolk sac cavity
Endometrium
Myometrium

Placental zone

Figure 4

Puppy
Amnion
                                    Chorioallantois
Allantoic cavity
Marginal hematomas

Parturition

PLATE 74

Figure 1. Cranial presentation of a puppy at delivery. Notice the protrusion of the chorioallantoic sac through the vulva. It is filled with allantoic fluid.

Figure 2. Caudal presentation of a puppy at delivery.

Using different colors, color the names and the structures indicated.

The average length of the gestation period (duration of pregnancy) in the bitch is 63 days. Extremes range from 59 to 70 days.

Some signs of impending parturition (the process of giving birth):
- Enlarged abdomen. Usually, but not always, an enlarged, relaxed vulva.
- Periodic discharge of clear mucus. Sometimes dried blood left over from the last heat.
- Increased size of mammary glands. Milk may be squeezed from the teats during during the last week of pregnancy.
- Body temperature drops to 98 - 99.5°F about 24 hours prior to parturition. Temperature should be taken every 12 hours.

Stage 1 of labor:
    Cervix dilates until it fills the caudal end of the vagina.
    Seclusion and nest building. Poor appetite.
    Increasing discomfort caused by uterine contractions. Rest, change position, walk, etc.

Stage 2 of labor - delivery of puppies:
    Labor contractions by ventral abdominal muscles create an abdominal press.
    Bitch will urinate, have a bowel movement, and possibly vomit.
    Puppy and fetal membranes are moved through the uterus, over the pubic brim, and through the birth canal (cervix. vagina and vulva). **Cranial presentation** occurs 60% of the time; **caudal presentation**, 40% of the time.
    The **chorioallantoic sac** (long dashes) filled with allantoic fluid emerges through the vulva or it may rupture first. The **amnionic sac** (short dashes) around the puppy will also rupture. These fluids provide lubrication for the passage of the puppy through the vagina. The puppy may or may not require assistance in delivery. With continuous licking, the bitch will rupture any intact fetal membranes and remove them from the puppy.

Expulsion of the placenta:
    The bitch pulls on the membranes and umbilical cord, pulling the placenta out. There is some bleeding. The canine placenta is deciduate, that is, there is some loss of maternal tissue at birth. The bitch eats the fetal membranes and the placenta.

Cesarean section (C-section), surgical delivery, is indicated when puppies are too large to pass through the pelvic opening or when they are in a position that prevents their passage from the uterus and through the birth canal. The large heads of fetuses of brachycephalic breeds usually require that the puppies be delivered by cesarean section.

Figure 1

Figure 2

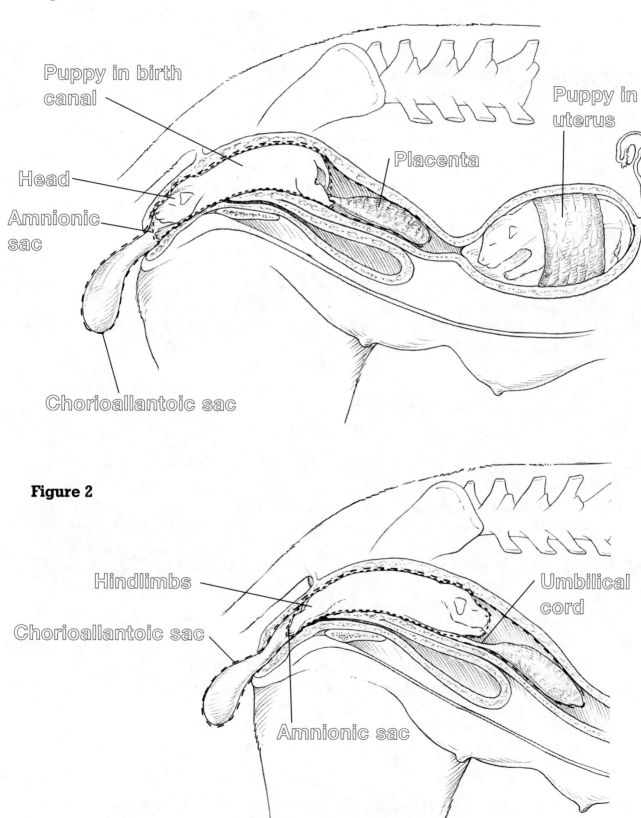

Canine Mammary Glands

PLATE 75

Figure 1. Ventral view of canine mammary glands
Figure 2. Diagrammatic drawing of a canine mammary gland.

Using different colors, color the names and the structures indicated.

There may be four to six pairs of mammary glands, but glands may be missing on either side. Frequently, opposite glands may be slightly staggered. This is a beneficial arrangement, since it provides better access for nursing puppies.

Mammary glands are modified sweat glands that develop to produce milk (lactate). **Secretory cells** lining **alveoli** produce milk. Star-shaped **contractile cells** (myoepithelial cells) surround each alveolus. **Lactiferous ducts** carry milk to **lactiferous sinuses**. **Papillary ducts** (teat canals) open on the end of the teat.

Late in pregnancy, mammary glands become larger as the secretory cells of alveoli produce more and more milk. In the final week or ten days, milk can be squeezed from the teats . The enlarged glands droop down, and opposite glands may touch one another.

All of the mammary glands lactate. When puppies begin to suckle (nurse), the mammary glands adjust to accommodate the number of puppies in the litter. Unneeded glands become swollen and firm, but the swelling soon decreases. Normally lactating glands become swollen and then decrease in size as they are suckled.

Suckling starts the "let-down reflex". Nervous stimulation by suckling causes secretion of a hormone (oxytocin from the pituitary gland). Oxytocin stimulates contractile cells around the alveoli to squeeze milk out into the lactiferous ducts.

The first milk produced, colostrum, has a laxative effect on the puppies. Colostrum also contains important antibodies that are ingested by the newborn puppy during the first day of its life. These antibodies provide protection against diseases for several weeks.

A firm, swollen, warm, possibly red mammary gland indicates mastitis, inflammation of a mammary gland caused by bacterial infection. Milk squeezed from the gland may have the thick appearance of pus, or it may be blood-streaked. A veterinarian should be consulted.

Mammary gland tumors, many cancerous, often occur in dogs. Lymph drainage from the cranial three glands on each side goes to the axillary lymph node; lymph drainage from the caudal two glands goes to the superficial inguinal lymph node (see Plate 65).

Figure 1

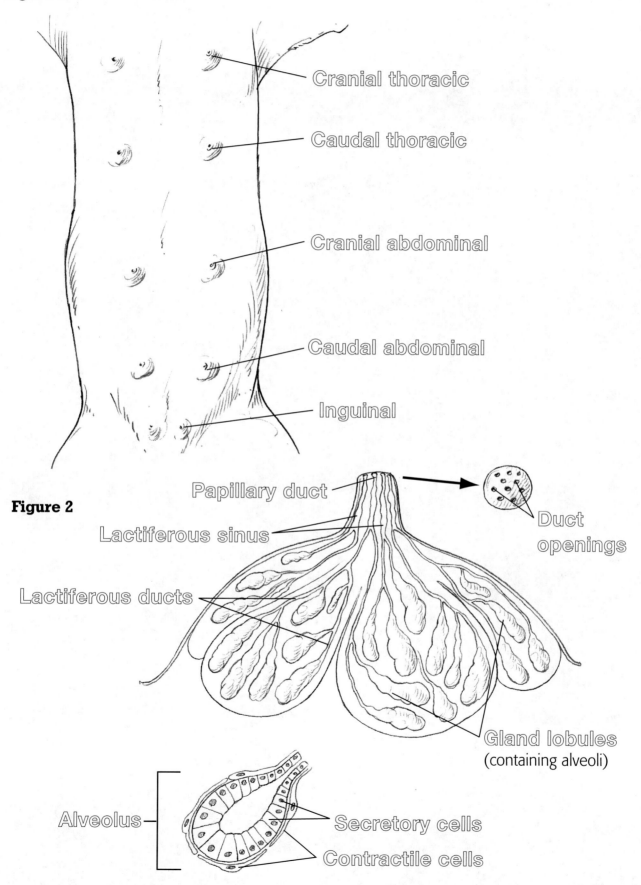

Cranial thoracic

Caudal thoracic

Cranial abdominal

Caudal abdominal

Inguinal

Papillary duct

Duct openings

Figure 2

Lactiferous sinus

Lactiferous ducts

Gland lobules
(containing alveoli)

Alveolus

Secretory cells

Contractile cells

Male Reproductive System

Genital Organs of the Dog

PLATE 76

Figure 1. Diagrammatic drawing of the male genital organs. Left lateral view.

Color the **boldfaced names** below and color the structures indicated on the plate.

1. **Deferent duct**
2. **Ureter**
3. **Bladder**
4. **Testicular vessels**
5. **Spermatic cord (within inguinal canal)**
6. **Prepuce**
7. **Penile bone**
8. **Long part of penile glans**
9. **Bulb of penile glans**
10. **Scrotum**
11. **Testis**
12. **Vaginal tunic**

13. **Ligament of tail of epididymis**
14. **Epididymis**
15. **Left cavernous body**
16. **Spongy body**
17. **Bulbospongiosus m.**
18. **Penile retractor muscle**
19. **Urethra**
20. **Prostate gland**

Figure 2. Section of right testis and epididymis.

Color the names and the structures indicated in different colors.

Each **testis** (Latin) (English, testicle; Greek, orchid) is suspended by a fold of peritoneum, the mesorchium, and enclosed by its continuaton, the **vaginal tunic**. Deep to the visceral part of the vaginal tunic, the dense fibrous connnective tissue **tunica albuginea** and its internally projecting septula support the testis. The **scrotum** is a pouch of skin, smooth muscle, fascia, and parietal vaginal tunic. The space between the visceral and parietal parts of the vaginal tunic is actually peritoneal cavity. Muscle in the scrotum and the cremaster muscles in the spermatic cord assist in regulating the temperature of the testicles by raising and lowering them from the body wall.

Sperm cells (spermatozoa) develop in **seminiferous tubules**. They pass through straight **tubules, testicular rete** (L., network) and **efferent ductules** into the **epididymal duct** in the **head of the epididymis**. As spermatozoa pass through the epididymal duct, they mature under the influence of secretions from the cells lining the duct. The terminal part of the epididymal duct in the **tail of the epididymis** and the first part of the deferent duct contain mature, motile spermatozoa with whip-like tails. The very muscular (smooth muscle) **deferent duct** continues up in the **spermatic cord** through the inguinal canal and terminates by opening into the prostatic part of the pelvic **urethra**. During ejaculation, each deferent duct propels spermatozoa and epididymal fluid to the urethra.

Figure 1

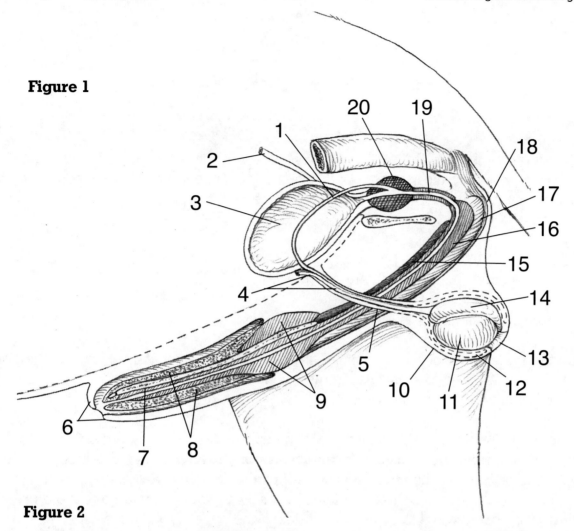

Figure 2

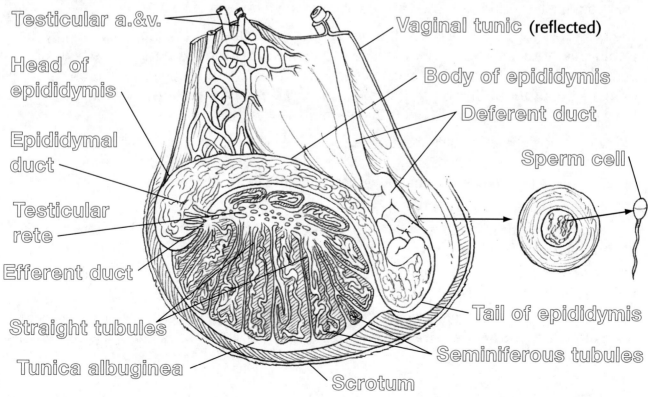

Testicular a.&v.

Vaginal tunic (reflected)

Head of
epididymis

Body of epididymis

Deferent duct

Epididymal
duct

Sperm cell

Testicular
rete

Efferent duct

Straight tubules

Tail of epididymis

Tunica albuginea

Seminiferous tubules

Scrotum

Prostate Gland. Penis

PLATE 77

Figure 1. Prostate gland. A. Dorsal view. B. Ventral view with urethra opened.
Figure 2. Relations of the erectile tissue bodies of the canine penis: roots of the penis, cavernous bodies, bulb of the penis, spongy body of the urethra, spongy body of the penile glans (L., glans penis).
Figure 3.
A. Cross section of bulb of glans penis.
B. Isolated penile bone (L., os penis. Also termed <u>baculum</u>).

Color the names and structures indicated on the drawings.

The **prostate gland** is the only accessory sex gland in the dog. Right and left lobes of the gland enclose the prostatic part of the **urethra**. Numerous ducts from secretory glandular units enter the urethra as it passes through the gland.

At the time of ejaculation, a mass of sperm cells and epididymal fluid is moved by muscular contractions of the **deferent ducts** and **ischiocavernous muscles** to the slit-like openings of the deferent ducts on each side of the **seminal hillock** in the dorsal wall of the prostatic urethra. This mass is moved toward the external urethral opening by contractions of the **urethral** and **bulbospongiosus muscles**. Then the prostate gland secretes, and the prostatic fluid and fluid from urethral glands is moved out, completing the formation of <u>semen</u>.

The two **roots** (or crura, L., legs) **of the penis** originate on the ischiatic tubers covered by the **ischiocavernous muscles**. They continue into the two **cavernous bodies** in the body of the penis. The **bulb of the penis** is situated between the two roots. It continues into the **spongy body of the urethra**. This expands into the **spongy body of the glans**. Arteries and veins of the penis are terminal branches of the internal pudendal vessels.

Erection of the penis is brought about by the complete filling of the erectile tissue bodies with blood. A complex sequence of arterial relaxation and interference with venous drainage caused by contractions of the muscles around the penis and the muscle of the vagina.

During sexual intercourse, it is mostly the extensive penile glans that enters the vagina. The bulb of the glans soon enlarges, causing a lock or <u>tie</u> with the vagina. As the male thrusts, the urethral opening of the penis is directed up toward the external opening of the cervix. The male and female may be "tied" for a long time - from 15 to 60 minutes. The male may change his position so that he faces away from the female.

At the end of intercourse, arterial flow returns to normal and muscles relax, permitting veins to open fully. The **two penile retractor muscles** contract, assisting the return of the penile glans into the **prepuce**.

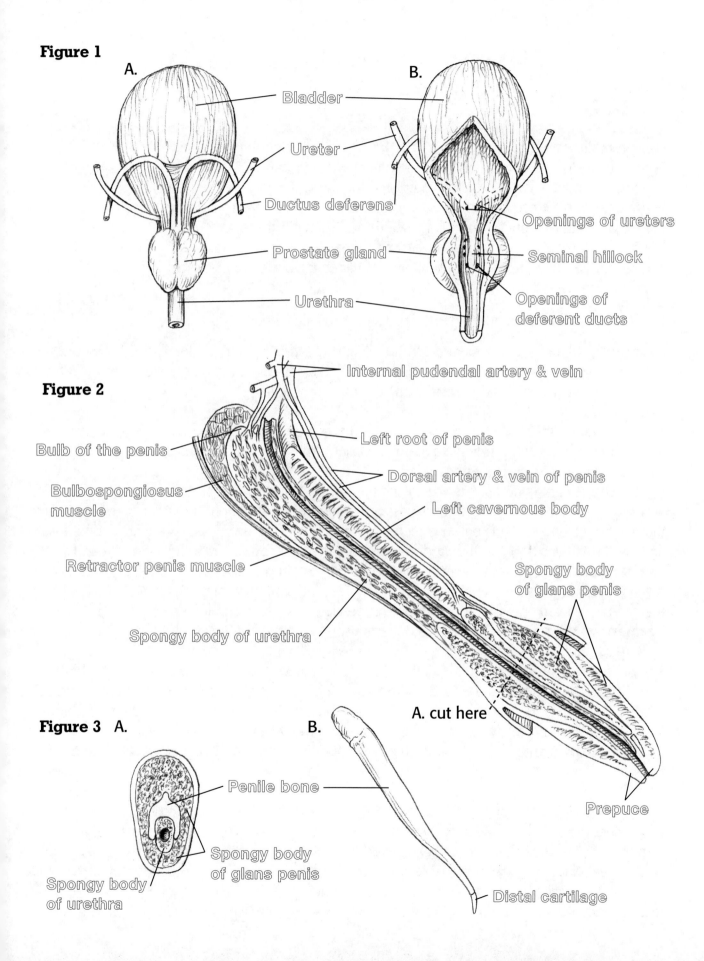

Figure 1

A.

B.

Bladder

Ureter

Ductus deferens

Prostate gland

Urethra

Openings of ureters

Seminal hillock

Openings of deferent ducts

Figure 2

Internal pudendal artery & vein

Bulb of the penis

Left root of penis

Bulbospongiosus muscle

Dorsal artery & vein of penis

Left cavernous body

Retractor penis muscle

Spongy body of glans penis

Spongy body of urethra

A. cut here

Prepuce

Figure 3 A.

B.

Penile bone

Spongy body of glans penis

Spongy body of urethra

Distal cartilage

Descent of the Canine Testes

PLATE 78

Diagrammatic drawings:
Figure 1. Testis and epididymis prior to entering inguinal canal. Extraabdominal part of the gubernaculum increases in volume to enlarge the inguinal canal and scrotum.
Figure 2. Loop formed by the epididymis and deferent duct enters expanded inguinal canal first.
Figure 3. Testis and epididymis within scrotum. Remnant of the gubernaculum persists as the ligament of the tail of the epididymis and proper ligament of the testis (not seen here). The parietal vaginal tunic (from the vaginal process) lines the scrotum; the visceral vaginal tunic covers the testis and epididymis.

Using different colors, color the names and structures indicated.

Each **testis** (plural = testes) begins as a swelling under a temporary middle kidney. As the developing testis begins to descend, the middle kidney regresses, but its duct becomes the duct of the **epididymis** and the **deferent duct**.

The **inguinal canal** is a potential space between the internal abdominal oblique muscle and the fibrous aponeurosis of the external abdominal oblique muscle. A slit in the aponeurosis is the superficial inguinal ring. The **gubernaculum** (L., helm) of jelly-like embryonic tissue (mesenchyme) grows and swells, expanding the **vaginal ring**, the inguinal canal and finally the **scrotum**. The descent of the testes is passive, forced by pressure from the growing organs around them. The gubernaculum is only a guide and does not contract even as it regresses. As the testis and epididymis descend into the **vaginal process**, they are covered with the inner **visceral vaginal tunic** that becomes continuous with the mesorchium (peritoneum suspending the testis). As each testis enters its compartment of the scrotum, the soft, regressing gubernaculum changes to the short, fibrous proper ligament of the testis between the testis and the epididymis and **ligament of tail of epididymis** that connects with the connective tissue of the scrotum.

The descent of the testes occurs in the last part of pregnancy and first several days after birth. The stimulus for descent of the testes is the hormone, testosterone, produced by cells within the testes. The testes are normally at the vaginal ring or into the inguinal canal at the time of birth. They should be completely descended into the scrotum by two weeks after birth. Due to the small size of the immature testes, they usually cannot be felt from the exterior until around six weeks after birth.

Retained testicle or cryptorchidism (Gr., kryptos, hidden, orchid, testis) can occur in dogs. The cryptorchid testis may be under the skin of the flank between the superficial inguinal ring and the scrotum. This has been termed a "high flanker". Two other locations are the inguinal canal or the abdominal cavity. Because of higher temperature, a retained testicle cannot produce spermatozoa, although it can still produce the hormone, testosterone. A monorchid (only one descended testicle) dog should not be used for breeding, since the abnormality is considered heritable.

Figure 1

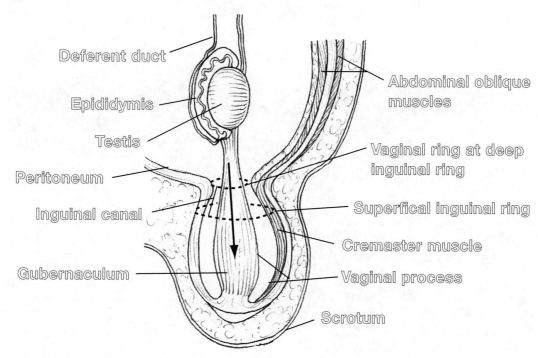

Deferent duct

Epididymis

Testis

Peritoneum

Inguinal canal

Gubernaculum

Abdominal oblique muscles

Vaginal ring at deep inguinal ring

Superfical inguinal ring

Cremaster muscle

Vaginal process

Scrotum

Figure 2

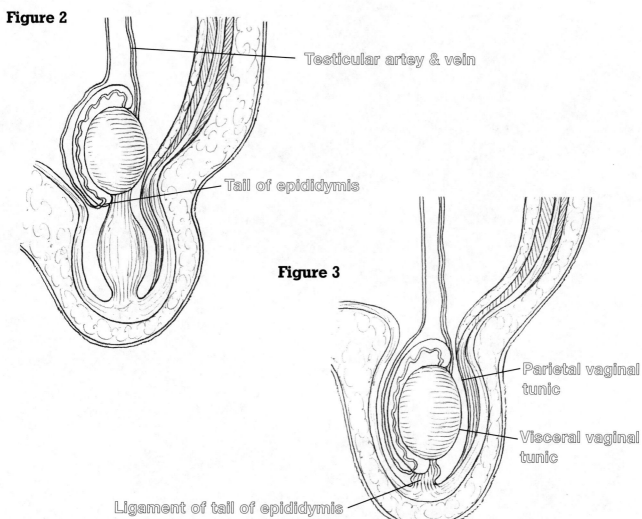

Testicular artey & vein

Tail of epididymis

Figure 3

Parietal vaginal tunic

Visceral vaginal tunic

Ligament of tail of epididymis

Nervous System

The Dog's Brain

PLATE 79

Figure 1. Dorsal view of brain.
Figure 2. Median section of brain.

Using different colors, underline the **boldfaced names** below and color structures indicated on the plate.

1. **Longitudinal fissure**
2. **Right cerebral hemisphere**
3. **Sulci** (grooves)
4. **Gyri** (convolutions)
5. **Cerebellum**
6. **Corpus callosum** (connects cerebral hemispheres)
7. **Septum pellucidum**
8. **Pineal gland**
9. **Medulla oblongata**
10. **Pons**
11. **Thalamus**
12. **Hypothalamus**
13. **Hypophysis cerebri or pituitary gland**
14. **Optic chiasm**
15. **Right optic nerve**
16. **Olfactory bulb**

The hypothalamus, pituitary gland, and pineal gland are parts of the endocrine system.

The three large parts of the brain are the cerebrum (with its two hemispheres), brain stem, and cerebellum. The brain stem consists of the pons, medulla oblongata, midbrain (mesencephalon), and between brain (diencephalon). The brain stem connects the cerebral hemispheres with the cerebellum and the spinal cord.

Figure 1

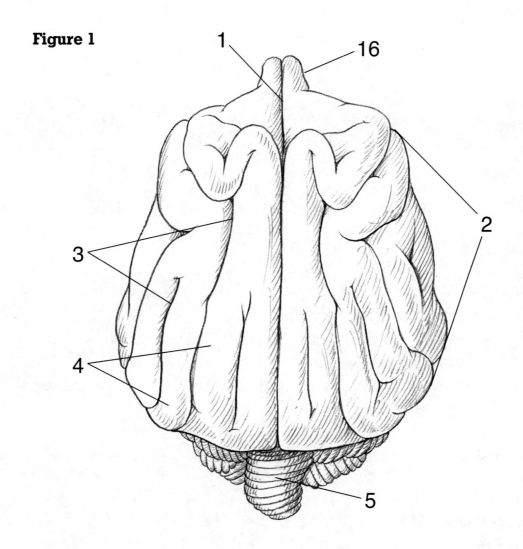

Figure 2

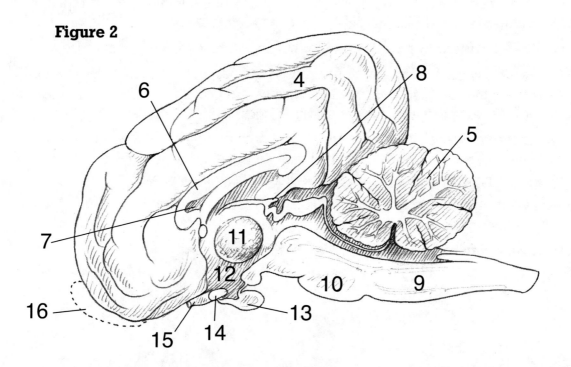

Cranial Nerves

PLATE 80

Ventral view of brain and cranial nerve roots.

In different colors, color the Roman numerals and the cranial nerves indicated on the plate.

CRANIAL NERVES and FUNCTIONS

I. Olfactory nerve - Sense of smell. Many small nerve fibers come from the mucous membrane of the two nasal fossae. They pass through openings in the cribriform plate of the ethmoid bone to the **olfactory bulbs**.

II. Optic nerve - Vision. Some nerve fibers coming from the retina of one eye cross over at the **optic chiasm** and continue into the optic tract of the opposite side.

III. Oculomotor nerve - Motor to several muscles around the eye. Parasympathetic fibers motor to smooth muscles within the eye.

IV. Trochlear nerve - Motor to trochlear muscle around the eye.

V. Trigeminal nerve - Sensory to face. Motor to muscles of mastication (chewing) and deep muscles of the head. Sensory to lower teeth. Lingual branch sensory for touch to the tongue.

VI. Abducent nerve - Motor to two muscles around the eye.

VII. Facial nerve - Motor to facial, eyelid and ear muscles. Its chorda tympani branch joins the lingual nerve and senses taste from the rostral 2/3 of the tongue. Parasympathetic fibers motor to lacrimal and salivary glands.

VIII. Vestibulocochlear nerve - Sensory for hearing and for motion and balance.

IX. Glossopharyngeal nerve - Motor to muscles of palate and pharynx. Senses taste and touch from the caudal 1/3 of tongue. Sensory to mucous membrane of palate and pharynx. Parasympathetic fibers to salivary glands.

X. Vagus nerve - Parasympathetic nerves to smooth muscle of cervical, thoracic, and abdominal viscera. Sensory to external ear. Sensory to laryngeal mucous membrane, and motor to laryngeal muscles via cranial and caudal laryngeal nerves.

XI. Accessory nerve - Motor to four shoulder muscles. Notice the main part of the nerve coming from the cervical spinal cord.

XII. Hypoglossal nerve - Motor to muscles of the tongue.

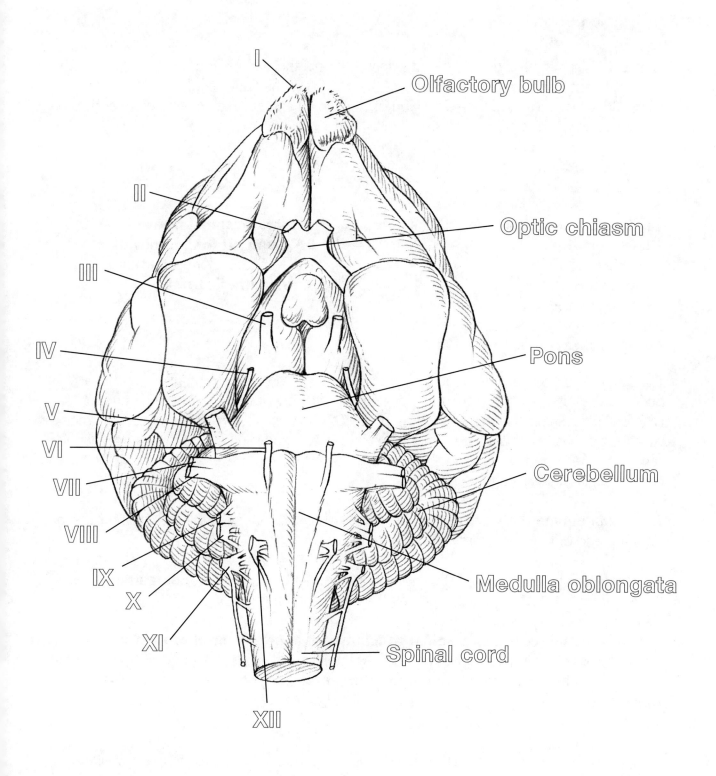

I

Olfactory bulb

II

Optic chiasm

III

IV

Pons

V

VI

VII

Cerebellum

VIII

IX

X

Medulla oblongata

XI

Spinal cord

XII

Spinal Cord and Spinal Nerves

PLATE 81

Figure 1. Diagrammatic dorsal view of spinal cord and spinal nerve roots.
Using different colors, color the names and the regions of the spinal cord.
Figure 2. Cross section of thoracic region of spinal cord and its relations to the vertebral canal and spinal nerve parts.

Underline **boldfaced names** below in different colors and color indicated structures on the drawing the same colors.

1. **Epidural space** (of vertebral canal)
2. **Dura mater**
3. **Spinal cord**
4. **Dorsal root**
5. **Spinal ganglion**
   (Nerve cell bodies and processes)
6. **Ventral root of spinal nerve**

7. **Thoracic spinal nerve**
8. **Communicating branches**
   (to and from sympathetic trunk)
9. **Sympathetic trunk**

The spinal cord continues from the medulla oblongata at the foramen magnum of the occipital bone, extending caudad to around the level of the intervertebral disc between L6 and L7. Differential development accounts for the presence of an eighth cervical spinal cord segment and variable relations of spinal cord segments to vertebrae. Caudal lumbar, sacral, and caudal segments of the cord lie more and more cranial to vertebrae of the same number. The spinal cord is longer in small dogs.

The **cauda equina** (L., horse's tail) is the collection of spinal nerve roots that extend caudad from the end of the spinal cord within the vertebral canal.

The diameter of the spinal cord is greatest at the **cervical** and **lumbar enlargements** where the nerve roots for the plexuses supplying the nerves of the limbs originate.

A sensory **dorsal root** (with its **spinal ganglion**) and a motor **ventral root** join to form a **spinal nerve**. The spinal nerve then divides into major dorsal and ventral branches. In the **thoracic** and **lumbar regions**, **communicating branches** connect with the **sympathetic trunk**. The latter is formed by a series of ganglia connected by nerves lying along the inner surface of the thoracic wall.

The dura mater, outermost meninx covering the spinal cord, is separated from the wall of the vertebral canal by an epidural space. This space contains some fatty tissue and a venous plexus. Spinal nerves pass through the meninges.

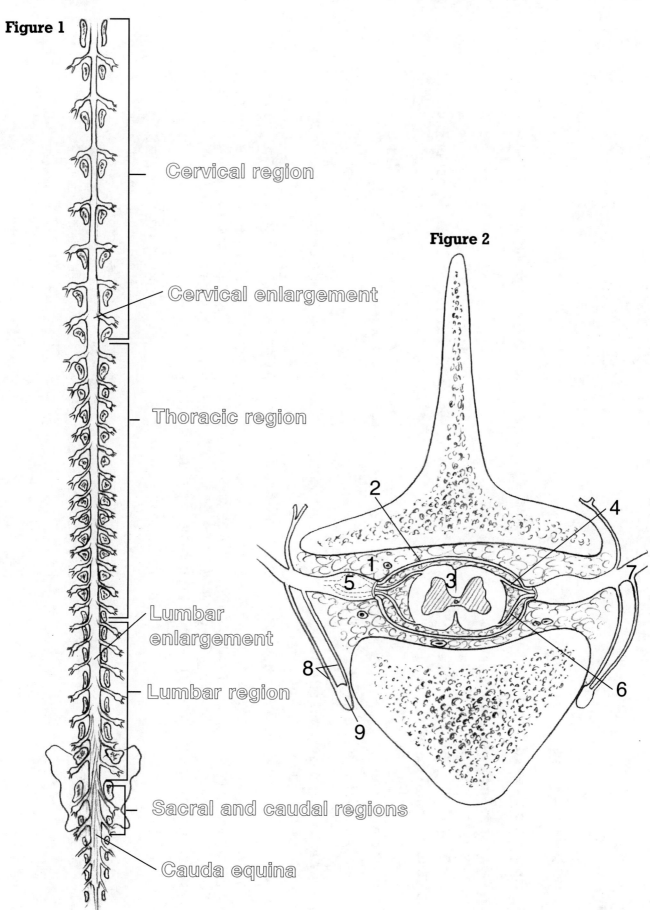

Figure 1

Cervical region

Cervical enlargement

Thoracic region

Lumbar enlargement

Lumbar region

Sacral and caudal regions

Cauda equina

Figure 2

2

4

1

5

3

7

6

8

9

Autonomic Nervous System

PLATE 82

Parasympathetic division - white; sympathetic division - black.

Underline the **boldfaced** names in different colors and color the structures indicated. Color the names on the plate.

1. **Parasympathetic nuclei** (collections of nerve cell bodies) in the brain stem. Sources of parasympathetic nerve fibers for cranial nerves III,VII, IX and X (**vagus nerve**)

2. **Cranial cervical ganglion** (collection of nerve cell bodies). Source of sympathetic nerve fibers supplying the head.

3. **Vertebral nerve**

4. **Sympathetic trunk and ganglia**

5. **Large sympathetic ganglia**

6. **Sympathetic nerves to thoracic, abdominal and pelvic organs**

7. **Vagal nerve branches to thoracic and abdominal organs**

8. **Pelvic nerves** - parasympathetic supply to pelvic organs.

The **vagus nerve** and **sympathetic trunk** are sheathed together as the vagosympathetic trunk that lies adjacent to the common carotid artery in the neck.

Both divisions of the autonomic nervous system are considered motor, but sensory nerve fibers course in autonomic nerves.

Nerve fibers from nerve cell bodies in the lateral grey horns of the thoracolumbar part of the spinal cord synapse with (pass nerve impulses to) nerve cells in sympathetic ganglia. Nerve fibers from cell bodies in the ganglia supply sympathetic innervation to the organs. Parasympathetic ganglia are within or on the organs that they supply with nerve fibers. Parasympathetic and sympathetic nerves usually supply the same organs, causing different responses:

ORGAN	PARASYMPATHETIC EFFECTS	SYMPATHETIC EFFECTS
Eye	Constriction of pupil	Dilation (expansion) of pupil
Lacrimal glands	Increased secretion	Decreased secretion
Salivary glands	Increased secretion	Decreased secretion
Heart	Decreased contraction rate	Increased contraction rate
Bronchi & bronchioles	Constriction	Expansion
Stomach & intestines	Increased motility and secretion	Decreased motility and secretion
Adrenal medulla	No effect	Secretion of epinephrine
Urinary bladder	Contraction	Relaxation

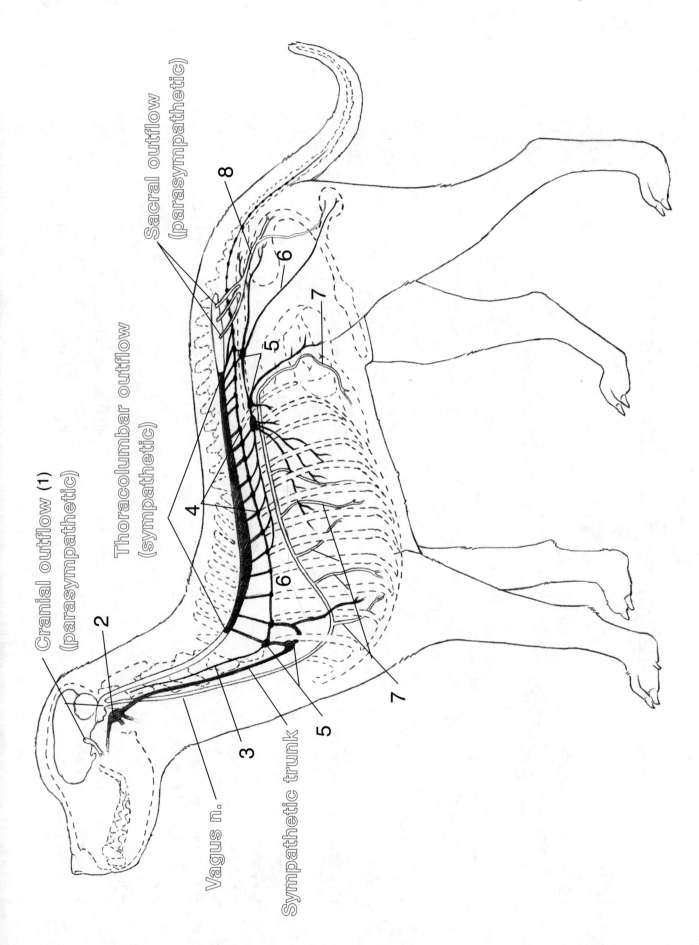

Cranial outflow (1)
(parasympathetic)

Thoracolumbar outflow
(sympathetic)

Sacral outflow
(parasympathetic)

Vagus n.

Sympathetic trunk

Meninges and Cerebrospinal Fluid

PLATE 83

Schematic drawing showing:

• Meninges (singular, meninx) - three membranes covering the brain and spinal cord.
• Main sites of production of cerebrospinal fluid (CSF), the **choroid plexuses**. CSF is also produced by the lining of the ventricles and brain tissue.
• Circulation of CSF (arrows) through the **ventricles** (communicating chambers of the brain), the central canal of the spinal cord and the **subarachnoid space.**
• Drainage of CSF through projecting **arachnoid granulations** into blood of a **venous sinus** within the **dura mater.**
• End of spinal cord and the **cauda equina** (L., horse's tail) formed by the last few spinal nerve roots.
• Sites for withdrawal of CSF (A) from the subarachnoid space and for injection of anesthetic into the **epidural space** (B), providing epidural anesthesia.

Underline the **boldfaced terms** in different colors and color the structures indicated by labels on the plate.

1. **Dura mater of cranial cavity** - blends with periosteum of cranial cavity; no epidural space.

2. **Dura mater of vertebral canal** - dense, fibrous outer meninx.

3. **Epidural space** (only in vertebral canal) - contains fatty tissue, vessels and nerve roots.

4. **Periosteum of vertebral canal**

5. **Arachnoid membrane** - delicate middle meninx.

6. **Subarachnoid space** (greatly enlarged here) - contains CSF. Crossed by spider web-like filaments extending from arachnoid membrane to pia mater.

7. **Pia mater** - vascular inner membrane covering brain and spinal cord; forms terminal filament at end of spinal cord.

8. **Cerebellomedullary cistern** - enlarged part of subarachnoid space; site for obtaining a sample of CSF.

9. **Interventricular foramen** (opening) - one each side; connects lateral ventricle in cerebral hemisphere with third ventricle.

10. **Third ventricle** - within midbrain.

11. **Choroid plexus of third ventricle** (Choroid plexus of lateral ventricle not seen here.)

12. **Fourth ventricle** - within medulla oblongata.

13. **Central canal of spinal cord** - continues caudal from fourth ventricle.

14. **Choroid plexus of fourth ventricle**

15. **Lateral aperture of fourth ventricle** - one of two exit foramina for CSF passing into subarachnoid space.

16. **Arachnoid granulations** - through which CSF passes into dorsal sagittal venous sinus.

17. **Dorsal sagittal venous sinus** - within dura mater.

CSF functions: **1.** Cushions brain and spinal cord. **2.** Transports nutrients, waste products, and regulatory substances. Hydrocephalus is an expansion of the ventricles filled with an excessive amount of CSF, exerting compression on the brain.

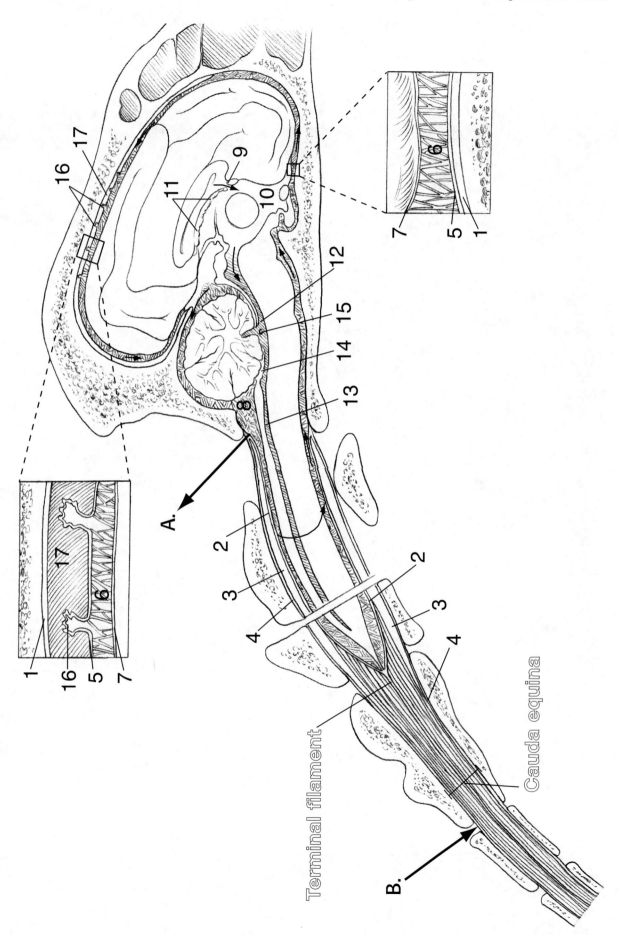

Terminal filament

Cauda equina

A.

B.

Endocrine System

Locations of Major Endocrine Organs

PLATE 84

In different colors, underline the **boldfaced names** of the endocrine organs listed and color the organs indicated on the plate.

ENDOCRINE ORGANS	HORMONES PRODUCED	TARGET ORGANS/TISSUES
1. Pineal gland	Melatonin	Sleep centers in brain
2. Hypothalamus	Releasing hormones	Anterior pituitary
	Oxytocin	Uterus, mammary glands
	Antidiuretic hormone (ADH)	Kidneys
3. Hypophysis cerebri (pituitary gland) **Anterior pituitary**	Thyrotropin	Thyroid gland
	Gonadotropins	Gonads: ovaries, testes
	Adrenocorticotropin	Adrenal cortices
	Somatotropin	Body's growing tissues
Posterior pituitary	Stores & releases oxytocin and ADH	See above
4. Thyroid gland - two lobes connected by an isthmus	Thyroxine & triiodothyronine	All tissues of body
	Calcitonin	Bone
5. Parathyroid glands two on each side	Parathyroid hormone (PTH)	Bone, intestines, kidneys
6. Stomach	Gastrin	Stomach, small intestine
7. Small intestine	Cholecystokinin; secretin	Gall bladder, small intestine
8. Pancreas	Insulin; glucagon	All tissues of body; liver, pancreatic islets,
	Somatostatin	gastrointestinal tract, anterior pituitary
9. Adrenal glands - cortex	Cortisol, aldosterone	All tissues of body, immune organs
- medulla	Epinephrine, norepinephrine	Muscular tissues, glands
10. Ovaries	Estrogens, progesterone	Female reproductive organs
Testes	Testosterone	Male repro. organs, muscle, skin
	Chorionic gonadotropin, estrogens	Female reproductive organs

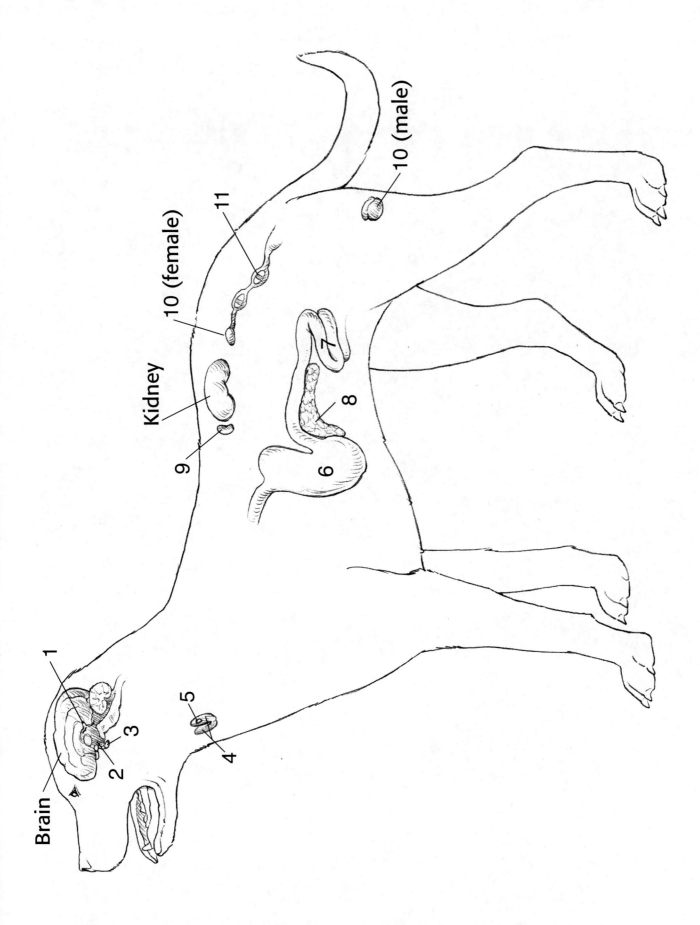

Brain

1

2

3

5

4

6

8

7

9

Kidney

10 (female)

11

10 (male)

Index

The plate numbers following the words refer to the narrative on the left page as well as the drawing(s) on the right page. All terms are listed under a main term. For example, to find Axillary artery, look under Artery (arteries), axillary.

NOTES

NOTES

NOTES